Reversal of Heart Disease

A FULL CIRCLE Book

Also available in Hindi Edition

हृदयरोग से मुक्ति

Reversal of Heart Disease

IN 5 EASY STEPS

Dr. Bimal Chhajer

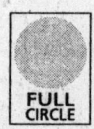

FULL
CIRCLE

REVERSAL OF HEART DISEASE
© Bimal Chhajer, 2003

First Paperback Edition, 2003
First Reprint, September, 2003
Second Reprint, February, 2004
Third Reprint, January, 2006

ISBN 81-7621-131-1

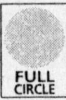

Published by FULL CIRCLE
J-40, Jorbagh Lane, New Delhi-110003
Tel: 24620063, 24621011 • Fax: 24645795
e-mail: fullcircle@vsnl.com • website:atfullcircle.com

Typesetting : SCANSET

J-40, Jorbagh Lane, New Delhi-110003
Tel: 24620063, 24621011 Fax: 24645795

Printed at Nutech Photolithographer, Delhi-110095

PRINTED IN INDIA
03/06/04/01/21/SCANSET/SAP/NP/NP

Foreword

I am very happy to write the foreword to the book *Reversal of Heart Disease* by Dr. Bimal Chhajer M.D.

Heart disease is born out of lack of knowledge and practical training. The most scientific treatment is understanding heart disease completely and bringing about adequate changes in life-style to solve it from the root. For a layman it is very difficult to read thousands of pages of information from the textbooks of cardiology and use them effectively in his daily life. The way that Dr. Chhajer and his team have explained and demonstrated the solution of heart disease is commendable as well as totally scientific.

Since I have joined the SAAOL Heart Program and reaped its benefits I would wish this knowledge to spread to the masses, so that people get real treatment and are able to avoid surgical treatment. During the course I received an earlier version of the manual and I know that the revised version will be a boon, to the general public who have heart disease or those who want to prevent it.

I strongly recommend this book to those who are not in a position to join the SAAOL Heart Program and follow the in-structions to reverse heart disease and reduce its risk factors.

I am sure the SAAOL Heart Program will help millions of heart patients not only in India but around the world.

Signed by

1. Dr. P.D. Padmakumar
2. Dr. P.S.B.R. James
3. Dr. A.D. Raman
4. Mr. Som Pal Varshney
5. Mr. U. Mukhopadhyay
6. Mr. B.S. Aswani

Signed by

7. Mr. Tilak
8. Mr. R. Singh
9. Mr. A.N. Chawla
10. Mr. K. Mahadevan
11. Mr. Suresh Gokuldas
12. Mr. R.L. Sharma
13. Ms. Lalita R. Patre
14. Mr. Bhushan Kumar
15. Mr. Shyamlal
16. Mr. A. Jayarajan
17. Mr. B.N. Wahi

18. Mr. K. Balasubramaniam
19. Dr. R.K. Bhatnagar
20. Mr. S.N. Purohit
21. Mr. Dinesh Chaurasia
22. Mr. Shreedharan
23. Mr. N. Damodaran Nair
24. Mr. A. Viswanathan
25. Mr. G.S. Sethia
26. Mr. A.S. Sarangi
27. Mr. Ashok Sen
29. Mr. Ramesh Chandra
    to 200

Note: Instead of getting the book recommended by known personalities I thought it would be better to get it recommended by my patients, i.e. participants of the SAAOL Heart Program. More than 200 of them penned similiar recommendations.

— Author

Acknowledgements

The writing of this book was a mammoth task and to complete the task a lot of help was required. This small chapter in the beginning is to formally thank those who helped me to bring out this book.

In the last sixteen years, after I started working in the field, everyone that I interacted with has somehow contributed to the book. All my patients who followed my program and achieved good results should be the first to be thanked. If they had not done what I wanted them to do — the SAAOL program would not have been successful. Their feedback, difficulties, their practical problems and blind belief in my arguments have all contributed to this book. Without them I would not have been able to develop such a wonderful program for heart patients. It was they who spread the program throughout the country and the world. They are part of the SAAOL Family which now has more than 5000 member families all over the world.

My wife Madhu, who has been my companion for the last thirteen years, is the second person on the list I would like to thank. It was her interaction with me that taught me many things in my life. Many of our ideas did not match. But the constant interactions taught me how to manage stress and interact without hurting others. As I learned practically, my talks on stress management became more vivid and practical. As we got more and more tuned to each other and understood Anekant — which says that no two people have the same ideas — my life became very smooth. This took about five years. She also had to bear the entire burden of looking after the family and to rear our children, especially as I started travelling a lot. She probably worked more than I did — to take care of the other end of family life. She complemented me wherever I lacked. She has been the force behind me in the fight against a system, which only promoted surgery and chemicals. Whenever I was feeling upset, it was she who stood like a rock beside me. She certainly deserves all the credit to make me what I am.

In order to remember and thank all those who helped me in my work, let me recollect them in sequence of time in the last sixteen years or so. This will assure that none of them is left out.

It was my Gurujee, late Acharya Shree Tulsi who encouraged me to take up the research that I started in 1986. He was in Delhi during that time. The Preksha System of Meditation and the brain behind this system, Acharya Mahaprajna, gave me the ideas that they could be a great tool to cure heart disease. In 1987, when I was doing my research in Lucknow — I got my firsthand experience in treating heart patients. I shall be eternally grateful to the owner of the Ashram, Sri Sudhir Sharma, assistants Renujee, Pandeyjee, Tewarijee etc. and my guide Dr. Tandon. They taught me yoga in the real sense.

When I came back to Delhi in 1989 I met Dharmanandjee, then assistant director of Adhyatma Sadhana Kendra, Mehrauli, through a friend, Mr. Dugar. Dharmanandjee — who after seeing my orientation and attachments in AIIMS (All India Institute of Medical Sciences, New Delhi) — never left me alone. For the next six years he supported me in whatever I needed to carry on my research in heart disease — money, infrastructure and personal training. Without him I would have never achieved many things in life. At AIIMS, there was Dr. Vijay Kumar, who now works in Chennai, gave me scientific back-up and was like a guide to me and more than a friend. Dr. K.S. Reddy, the most known person in Preventive Cardiology in India, the two Dr. Manchandas at AIIMS — in Physiology and Cardiology, Dr. Usha Sachdeva, Dr. SC Mahapatra take the credit for directly training me at AIIMS. In 1995 I resigned from AIIMS. I am happy that the treatment project that we started there has now grown and the research results have been published recently. I would have been happier if they had not diluted the food restrictions to suit the patients and improved results.

It was during a major conference at AIIMS in 1990 organised by Dr. Reddy that I had a direct contact with Dr. Dean Ornish's group. Dr. Larry Scherwitz, the co-investigator in Dean Ornish's study was at the conference and on my request he organised a workshop on Dean Ornish's way at Delhi. Two years from then I attended a workshop with Dr. Ornish. Since then, I learned everyday from his projects — his books, research papers, his cassettes. The only variation from Dean Ornish's program was the Indianisation in cooking, addition of a very good stress management program, use of Preksha system (which is definitely a better system than the simple meditation that Ornish uses) and a long term friendly follow-up with my patients. Dr.Ornish has remained my inspiration all through and my strong conviction in his research has led to the development of the SAAOL Heart Program.

In 1995, I organised an International Conference on 'Lifestyle and Health' at AIIMS. This gave me a boost in my program. I started thinking better and for the community at large. During the conference I got immense support from Dr. Baid, Mr.Vinay Maloo and Sri Dharmanand, which I cannot forget.

When I found a lot of resistance and red tapism to promote my ideas at a Government institution like AIIMS, I decided to quit and start on my own. I did not have any facilities, funds or infrastructure. But my wife was a source of great support and my brother, Kamal, provided me with the funds. SAAOL was thus born. I have never looked back thereafter.

During the early days of inception of SAAOL, I had great difficulties in convincing my patients to join the program. The more I tried to convince, the more I learned. Those who believed me, got results and thus more patients were introduced to me. Those who joined me in the first one year were probably very close to me, as I felt they joined the program without a lot of credibility but with the conviction that this young doctor is talking sense. They are still with me and I continue seeing many of them on a monthly basis. They deserve a lot of thanks, for depending on me and supporting the program in its early stage.

All through the last few years at SAAOL (1995 to 2002) we, my colleagues and I changed a lot in the SAAOL Heart Program. We kept making the program more and more practicable and easy, without compromising on the parameters. We developed a new system of zero oil cooking, a complete system of stress management and a better delivery system to the patients. We asked the old groups to meet the new groups — to tell them what they did and what is possible. This gave a big boost to the program and convinced the new groups that it was possible to improve. I am really indebted to those members who shared their experiences in the get-togethers which I held on the third day of all my programs. Many of them wrote about their experiences and I have included those experiences in the twelfth chapter of this book. I am sure they will also imbibe enthusiasm in the readers who wish to reverse their heart ailment.

Those who worked with me in the last four years have also helped me to develop the program. The resident doctors Dr. Arijit Chakravorty, Dr. Sunil Sikand, Dr. Nehal Ahmed, Dr. Vishal Sharma, Dr. Kapil Sharma and Dr. Rajeev Sharma worked with me and each one of them have directly and indirectly helped me to establish the program. Nehal and Vishal have stayed for a longer time and have contributed more in terms of inputs. Amongst the dieticians, two ladies who I most admire and thank are Yamini and Veenu — both worked with us for more than two years and helped me in my last popular zero oil cookbook, *Food for Reversing Heart Disease*. Ruchi, Anu, Smriti, Priyanka and Anjana also worked with SAAOL and in helped our work.

Among the support staff and my other colleagues were Sonia Wadhwa (now Mrs. Pradeep) and Deepti Chaudhary, who had been of exceptional help to me. They stood beside me all the time whenever we required them. Sonia left us after marriage and Deepti still works with us shouldering a lot of our work.

Others who worked to contribute to this book, little or more, are Meghrajee and Kishore (our accountants), Geeta, Meenakshi, Monika Narula, Sagar, Amit, Sarabjeet, Chhotelal, Bhujram, Sanjay, Tarkeshwar Babu and some others whose names I may be forgetting now. I thank all of them from my heart.

So far as writing this book is concerned, without Sudheer and Ajit it would not have been possible. Sudheer typed all the pages of the book and edited it a few times in the last one year. He would sit till midnight sometimes though his duty finished at 7 p.m. I admired his patience. Ajit, my nephew, who joined me about 2 years back had taken over much of my work and thus it gave me more time to work on the book. He also helped me a lot in getting the first edition of the first edition of the book printed. I cannot forget his contribution.

Four people who helped me in the camps that I conducted in the last few years were Mr. Jain, Mr. Trehan, Mr. Arun Kumar and Mr. L. K. Jha. They are all yoga experts who immensely contributed to the development of the SAAOL Heart Program. I remain indebted to them.

This book got corrected a few times, and Mr. Deepak Dalal, our Mumbai co-ordinator, whom I trust most, has been responsible for the major corrections. He meticulously went through all the pages and corrected them. Others who corrected the book were Dr. Airi, Dr. D'souza and Mr. A.S. Yadav. I must express my gratitude to Sagar who designed the original book so well.

I would also like to pay my regards to my parents, who were my source of inspiration. Wherever I worked, I always remembered that their blessings are with me, and that contributed to my good work. My sister Kabita, was also a psychological help, as I know she is the one who really cared for me. My two brothers and their wives — they stay in Hyderabad and Chennai — had also been a source of energy for me. Their love and trust in my work has given me a boost. My children Gaurav and Garvit gave me a source of unending energy that allowed me to work very hard and travel throughout India to spread the message of SAAOL.

My life has been affected and influenced by a lot more people, who I fail to recall at this moment. But I always thank them in my mind — whenever I remember them.

I know all these people will be happy when the revised edition of the book hits the stands and becomes an instrument for helping millions of people from unnecessary suffering and the ordeal of undergoing heart attacks or surgery.

Lastly I would like to thank FULL CIRCLE Publishers, especially Poonam and Shekhar Malhotra, for encouraging us and publishing the revised edition of the book.

Dr. Bimal Chhajer

Contents

Section 1

Introduction

Contents

Some books are to be tasted, others to be swallowed, and some few to be chewed and digested.

— BACON

Is reversal possible?

Reversal of heart disease? A very common query that I have come across in the last few years from everybody — colleagues, doctors, patients, friends and visitors.

Thousands of times I have been asked how is it possible to 'Reverse'? People have expressed surprise about the theory of reversal of coronary heart disease. They have been doubtful about what they have not heard so far.

Well, I wonder why there should be a doubt when it is pure common sense, that something that is deposited can be withdrawn as well. Bank deposits can be withdrawn, deposits on a floor can be removed, buildings can be demolished, deposited calcium from the bone can be removed in old age, and stains on shirts can be removed.

Then why not the deposits inside the arteries of the heart? Why does this common sense seem so absurd when it comes to the cholesterol deposits in the arteries of the heart? Why is reversal of heart blockages not possible?

The answer is, "It was not known previously." With the worsening life-style, people have not seen this happening often. The doctors and cardiologists have not tried to remove the deposits, as they never directed people to remove the causes of the deposits. Deposition was going on and on for the last few decades, nobody tried to put the car in the reverse gear.

> The art of medicine consists of amusing the patients, while nature cures the disease.
> — Voltaire

In science something new is discovered everyday. Events when proved beyond doubt are accepted as facts, though earlier they were not accepted. Today the fact that blockages inside the heart supply-tube can be re moved is fully accepted. It is a part of the books on cardiology now.

The idea of bringing out this book is to inform laymen who are not doctors, that reversing this common and dreadful disease is absolutely possible. All you need to do is to understand the disease, to know how the disease has grown and do exactly the opposite of what has led to the blockages.

Genius is the ability to reduce the complicated to the simple.

SAAOL — the real treatment of heart disease

Heart disease is one of most common and fatal diseases the modern times. Fifteen years ago it was believed that once it develops in a person it can only progress. It was a continuously progressive disease. And we also saw that the number of patients were increasing in the last few decades. There was no solution. A large number of people started having heart attacks and half of them died even before reaching the hospital.

If you ever try to analyse, you will come to know that the disease is due to the slow but steady deposit of fatty material — cholesterol and triglycerides inside the arteries of the heart and we have allowed them to grow with our modern life-style. The food with fats and oils that we are eating today cannot be utilised as we have stopped exerting physically. The unused and extra fat, with the help of factors like stress/tension of modern life, smoking habits and so on, has no option other than to get slowly deposited inside the body and the heart arteries — causing heart disease. Somehow

> Your doctor is the second most important person taking care of your health. You're the first.
> — HARVARD MEDICAL SCHOOL HEALTH LETTER

these simple facts were ignored over the years and we gradually got engulfed in an ever-growing and ever-killing trap of heart disease.

The good news is that by bringing about small but informed changes in our life-style we cannot only prevent the growth of the heart disease but also reverse it. This would mean, in other words, that it is now possible to remove the fat and cholesterol deposits which obstruct the flow of blood to the heart muscles.

Medical research has now proved beyond any doubt (supplemented with angiographic proofs) that heart disease reversal is possible only with a combination of the knowledge of medical science and art of yogasana, cooking, stress management, meditation and use of common sense. And thus the term, SAAOL (the Science And Art Of Living).

Allopathy, the modern medical science, has the knowledge about the human body, knowledge about the cholesterol deposits, what is the structure of the chemical called triglycerides, which foods contain more cholesterol and triglycerides, how many calories does the body require, what exercises have to be offered to the body and so on. Without this knowledge we cannot know the disease and its causes. Without its modern medical gadgets like ECG, stress test (TMT), cholesterol test and so on, it will be impossible to prove the reversal. Being a medical doctor I have made use of the good elements of allopathic science to cure heart disease.

Allopathic medicine also has its drawbacks. It does not speak about stresses of life, which is one of the most important factors for causing heart disease and heart attacks. It has completely failed to measure and quantify stresses. It also offers no solution except for sleeping pills and anti-anxiety tablets. It knows that the human mind is the site of all stresses but is still to accept completely that it is actually possible to control the mind

> God heals and the doctor takes the fee.
> — FRANKLIN BEN

(brain) through psychotherapy and meditation.

Though allopathy talks about cholesterol and fats, and says that they cause the blockage — it lacks common sense about how to prepare food without them. While exercise is recommended, the ancient Indian art of yogasana — the safest exercise for heart patients — has not been adopted.

The irony is that the allopathic science has also forgotten common sense. Instead of solving the real problems that cause heart disease it has ventured into abnormal and unreasonable methods called Bypass Surgery and Angioplasty. Doctors without solving the real causes have been completely dependent on more and more drugs, and only on drugs. (I will point out how and who for their selfish motives, diverted the allopathic science over the years). This is where I have not adopted the allopathic science. I have only used the goodness of modern science.

We, at SAAOL, on the other hand, chose all the best of the art of living to treat heart patients and combined them with the best of allopathic science and put them together. This combination has been developed over the last sixteen years of intense research at King George's Medical College, Lucknow; All India Institute of Medical Sciences (AIIMS), New Delhi and in the whole of India, as a part of development and spread of the SAAOL Heart Program. During this long period, we have validated the program on more than 5000 patients. In the process of spreading it we have indirectly helped more than a million people to prevent and reverse heart disease. This book is the outcome of our years of extensive research and development.

SAAOL started as a small organisation in September, 1995, in Lajpat Nagar, Delhi and today it has spread to all parts of India. It has spread mainly through word of mouth. Those who saw results inspired others. Those who appreciated the theory disseminated the information. We called our patients' families 'SAAOL Family' and the culture as 'SAAOL Culture'. It has now become a universal word. Today we have SAAOL families in every corner of the country, and in more than thirty countries of the world.

We have already brought out a food book called *Food for Reversing Heart Disease*, a journal called '*Heart Talk*' and another book called *Understanding Heart Disease*. This publication is the latest in the series.

Any interference with nature is damnable. Not only nature but also the people will suffer.

— ANAHARIO

Progress or failure of cardiology

The growing incidence of coronary heart disease (or angina) has led to the development of more and more artificial and unnatural therapeutic approaches, new drugs, coronary care units, bypass surgeries, angioplasties etc. The results of these, though sometimes dramatic, find limited applications as the number of heart patients grossly outnumber the established capacities of hospitals, and because of high cost involvement and their temporary effect. What I found is that none of these new and latest hi-technology developments of modern medical science are directed to the real cause of the problem. These over publicised, artificial, technically unreasonable and expensive treatments may have given lots of funds to doctors to develop big hospitals and cardiac centres, but for patients there has been little or no long term gain, as nothing has been done to solve heart problems from the root.

As per the estimates, in the year 2001 there were more than 50,000,000 people suffering from coronary heart disease in India, and if we go by the exaggerated estimate only a total number of 50,000 people could get bypass surgeries done

> A single fact is worth a shipload of argument.
> — A PROVERB

and as many could get angioplasties done in India. Even if both grow at the same rate of 10% per year the difference is going to increase dangerously. With only 100,000 people getting these interventions, the estimated cost is nearly one thousand crore rupees. What about the rest of the people? The re-blockages? Think of the medical maintenance therapy for those who do not want an intervention or cannot afford it (total number being about 4,99,00,000). Most of these patients are spending over Rs.1000/- a month on a regular basis for maintenance therapy, yet they may never attain a permanent cure even after years of therapy. More so even the way the number of heart patients is growing the total number is going to reach 100,000,000 (100 million or 10 crore) heart partients in India by the year 2010.

People think that cardiology has progressed, based on the commercial success of the big cardiac hospitals. Any person with a little common sense should understand that even in this era of the so called progress of cardiology, if the number of patients is growing, where is the progress. Success of a treatment system must lead to the reduction of the suffering population.

> Somebody commented the other day, "Doctor, the cardiology department is the most progressive branch of medical science, compared to other branches."
> I asked, "What kind of progress did you see?"
> He observed that so many cardiology, bypass surgery, angioplasty hospitals are coming up every day. So many new techniques are being developed.
> I asked him a very simple fact, "What about the number of patients?"
> "They are growing at a faster speed. Every house seems to have a heart patient, because of this the queues in front of these cardiac hospitals are also growing," the reply came.
> I asked him, "If the number of patients is growing, do you think of it as success or failure?"

This is what has happened with India's success in eradicating small pox or polio. We don't see small pox at all and hardly any polio patients these days. That is success. But how can one call it a success or progress when the number of patients is growing?

I would rather say that the surgeons and intervention-cardiologists must have progressed (may be financially or status wise) but modern allopathic cardiology has completely failed. The status of cardiology has gone down and the condition of the patients has gone down. The big buildings are the sign of financial success of the business activities of these hospitals and the up-coming new techniques are mainly an effort to avoid the failures or complications of the prevailing techniques.

The real solution has always been eluding us, as nobody wanted to solve the root causes of heart disease. Hospitals, bypass surgeons and angioplasty specialists have financial and academic reasons to promote their system. They have never looked beyond. Medical companies and cardiologists have always promoted drugs and maintenance and emerg-ency therapy. The result has been that no real and permanent solution has ever been seriously thought of or offered.

SAAOL (Science and Art of Living) is a unique approach which not only looks into the causes of the dreadful coronary heart disease but also tries to present a long-term solution. The aim is to control all the cardiac risk factors together and prevent/cure the disease from the root. It has combined the best of the knowledge of medical science and the best of the ancient and common art of living. The results over the past decade have shown us that this cannot only stop the progress of the blockages but also reverse it. In the face of a complete failure of the hard-core medical cardiology, which has failed to deliver the goods because its approach was wrong, a perfect

> The men the American people admire most extravagantly are the most daring liars; the men they detest most violently are those who try to tell them the truth.
>
> — H.L. MENCKEN

combination of science and art was the real need.

A combination of a guided life-style, education, yoga, meditation, stress reduction programs and dietary-cum-cooking training is what SAAOL has offered to its participating patients. The results of the system have gradually spread, as more and more people followed it and got cured.

Today there is a great amount of awareness all over India and abroad amongst heart patients and those who want to prevent the disease, about this non-invasive solution.

I do not think that the measure of a civilisation is how tall its buildings of concrete are, but rather how well its people have learned to relate to their environment and fellowmen.

— SUN BEAR, CHIPPEWA TRIBE

Why heart patients are increasing in number?

It is astonishing that heart disease (otherwise known as angina, coronary heart disease, coronary artery disease, ischaemia or ischaemic heart disease) is very common even though the reasons of the disease are very well-known. Not only is it very common but the number is also growing at a very high rate, in spite of so many doctors practising cardiology and so many heart hospitals being opened to tackle the problem. What could be the reason?

The population of this country is about 100 crore (1000 million) today and as many as 5 crore people seem to have a heart problem. About 30 crore people living in India in this modern era have the risk of developing a heart disease in the near or distant future. Another bad trend is the lowering of the age of the suffering population.

> Facts are facts and will not disappear on account of your likes.
>
> — JAWAHAR LAL NEHRU

More and more people below the age of 40 are getting a heart disease. The reason for this dangerous trend is now known. It is the wrong life-style.

It is also apparent that the younger population is having a very wrong life-style so as to create the heart blockage in 10 to 15 years compared to 30-40 years in the past. As usual they now do things faster !

If we look at the causes of the disease, it is due to excessive deposits of cholesterol and fat (triglycerides) inside the tubes that supply blood to the heart muscles. Excessive intake and less utilisation of these two fatty materials are the main reasons for the deposits. Factors aggravating the blockages are — excessive stress, lack of exercise, smoking, high blood pressure and high blood sugar. Almost all of them are related to our life-style. Whatever we do, if we do not remove the causes of blockage, the disease and the deposits grow.

The irony is that modern medical science has not tried to remove the causes of the disease. Not only have they overlooked the disease etiopathology but they have also exploited people and taken advantage of the disease. Without removing the reasons which lead to deposits of cholesterol and fat, they have taught people to postpone the problem with the use of continuous medication. Another group of doctors and cardiologists have started temporary techniques like angioplasty and bypass surgery. They have tried to intervene the blockage by invasive procedures which are lucrative to them, without caring to cure the disease from the root. People are also falling into this trap, as there is nobody to give them the knowledge or explain the temporary nature of the treatment. The temporary relief from angina, after an artificial scare caused before the surgery or angioplasty, makes them happy but the disease remains unattended. Both ways the number of diseased persons is growing.

Most people would rather die than think, and they do.

— GEORGE BERNARD SHAW

Why people do not take care even after getting heart disease?

The idea that has been passed on to people at large is that either they need an expensive and mutilating surgery or they have to take some tablets to get relief. As the disease grows (in the absence of proper life-style change), the condition goes from bad to worse and the patients suffer from a fatal condition called heart attack.

Now there is a huge scare amongst people about heart disease. But they do not know what to do. They only know a little bit and that too is mostly incorrect. When they come to know about the disease, they try to follow as much as they know but as their information base is not correct and adequate most people do not get the results or relief. When the results do not come, they give up. Then they see cardiologists, get medicines as a treatment and get some relief. So they stick to them and as these doctors do not have the time to explain to their patients about life-style, the patients do not understand the importance. I often feel that doctors are now working more as pharmacologists as far as heart disease is concerned. They have not promoted health but instead are promoting medical companies.

The only hope I can see for the future depends on a wiser and braver use of reason, not a panic flight from it.

—F.L. Lucas

What should be done now?

The need of the day is practical education along with proper training to the patients. This responsibility actually lies with doctors and cardiologists. These are the people who should have promoted a healthy life-style and scientific education. But they have failed to do this duty almost completely.

I do not want to blame only doctors for this. Our medical system's orientation has not been correct. Cardiologists are too busy to give this kind of explanation. Due to the increasing number of patients they are only left with time for writing prescriptions and solving emergencies (when blocks are allowed to grow the emergency is sure to come). The commercial nature of their unidirectional private practice is also to be blamed for this attitude. Maybe some of them consider it below their dignity to talk about food, yoga and exercise to their patients.

The future of cardiology lies not in the present superfluous high technology operations but on treating heart patients by advocating appropriate low technology life-style changes. Though this technique is low in technology and easy to deliver, it is fool-proof, long term and most effective. The number of heart patients can only be reduced by changing the life-style and this advice has to come from doctors in a very scientific, practical and user-friendly way. Cardiologists should come out of their selfish shell and open up to the patients and advise them what is best for them.

I am not completely against the administration of medicines or surgery. Medicines may have to be administered till such time as patients reverse their disease and besides some side effects of these chemicals, there is nothing to lose. But to my mind almost all these high technology surgeries and interventions (bypass surgery and angioplasties) would not be required in future if all the suggested life-style changes can be incorporated in the patient's life.

I have my doubts about making it possible in a great way, not because it is difficult for patients to change their life-style but because the cardiology group will try to continue utilising their hospitals and facilities, which have been developed with considerable investments.

> If I go to heaven, I will take my reason with me.
> — R.G. Ingersoll

I am, at least, happy that gradually there is an increasing awareness against these surgeries and towards changing life-styles of the patients. Many like-minded cardiologists are now encouraging patients to change their food habits and are advising them to exercise regularly. Ultimately the patients will realise the easier and most appropriate way to handle their disease.

To a greater extent most of us are willing to accept that today's disorders of overweight, heart disease, cancer, blood pressure and diabetes are by and large preventable. In this light, true health insurance is not what one carries on a plastic card, but what one does for oneself.

My experience in treating heart patients and developing a program for reversing heart disease

As a part of my research in the first ten years of my career after passing my MBBS in 1986 from Kolkata, I gradually started advocating more and more life-style changes to heart patients. Initially I was using only yoga and meditation to treat heart patients; I found them effective but insufficient. I used mostly yoga in my treatment protocol during my research work for MD at King George's Medical College, Lucknow till 1989. Gradually I started telling them about avoiding fats and oils. This added power to my treatment.

When I started my research at the All India Institute of Medical Sciences (AIIMS) in 1990, I proposed a three pronged attack which included yoga, diet and stress management as a treatment mode. By then the results of the treatment had become very fast and visible. Patients were improving considerably. After training with Dr. Ornish and experiencing with my own patients at

In science we must be interested in things, not in persons.
— MARIE CURIE

AIIMS, I included educating the patients and exercise in my program. I realised that if patients do not know about heart disease and the logic behind each component of the program, they tend to make mistakes and gradually drift away from the program.

The final program was developed after I resigned from AIIMS and started the SAAOL Heart Program. While at AIIMS I was telling my patients only to avoid oil and cholesterol. They would definitely do so as they were under tremendous pressure to cure their heart disease, but the food was tasteless. As soon as their health improved, there was an urge to eat normal food, which was cooked with oil and fat. Since I was looking for a permanent treatment I could not afford to allow this. The only solution was to make the food tasty.

As the saying goes, where there is a need and urge, there will be an invention. This urge in 1995-96 made me ask, "Why can't we make food tasty without oil?" Experiments started and gradually evolved into a complete system of cooking tasty food without a drop of oil. The food part was almost solved.

As my patients grew under the SAAOL Heart Program, we kept a close watch on their practical difficulties and adherence levels. The yoga program was gradually refined and made more effective. In every camp we collected feedback from our patients (from all areas of India — north, south, east and west) and incorporated it into our program. The results gradually improved. Now I have treated more than 5000 heart patients by the SAAOL Heart Program with tremendous success all over the country.

It is hard to fail but it is worse never to have tried to succeed. In this life we get nothing save by effort.

— THEODORE ROOSEVELT

Why this book?

As I found that the SAAOL Heart Program had created a tremendous awareness all over the country and the continent (we have held the program in Thailand), I realised that I cannot directly train more patients as the demand is growing beyond my capacity. I expanded my capacity and spread the training program to all the Metro cities. Then I asked myself, "What is my capacity?" I realised that compared to five crore heart patients in India, my capacity was very limited. There were a large number of people who could not avail of my program for want of time or money. Thus the idea of writing a book, rather a manual, came to my mind.

I know a doctor is a doctor. You can't give a medical book to a patient and expect him to write a prescription for himself. But whatever can be done is better than doing nothing. If I can directly help 2000 patients in a year, the rest 4.99 crore have a right to get as much as possible rather than getting nothing.

I know lacs of people who suffer from heart disease and are trying to do something with the help of may be a yoga teacher, a friend or another book. But with half-hearted efforts the results are not forthcoming and they are continuing to suffer. As I explained, doing a part of the program would help but would not be adequate. Replacing ghee with another oil is not good enough. Just walking or consuming fruit juices is grossly inadequate as a treatment. If someone has to really reverse he/she has to know every aspect of the treatment. This is another important reason for my coming out with this book. I wanted to inform a heart patient about everything that he may need to know in his own language.

This book is not only meant for those who have already developed heart disease (which effectively means blockage of more than 70%) but also for those who have one or the other risk factor for developing heart disease. These risk factors may be high blood pressure, bad food habits, overweight, diabetes, high stress job or family life, or high blood cholesterol or a family history of heart disease.

All these people must learn that they have, in all probability, started developing blockages. May be the percentage is just 10-50% but that is sufficient enough for following this book. I would presume that there are about 30 crore such people who fall in this category. This book is going to be of tremendous help for this very large populace.

I feel this book is the need of billions of people and all of them have a right to know their disease and understand the remedy. I do not want to deprive them of this knowledge which can save them from severe suffering, a heart attack, a bypass surgery or an angioplasty. Let the knowledge spread. My efforts of the last one and a half decades would reap more harvest and I would consider myself blessed, if the lives of people are saved as a result of the knowledge contained in this book.

He, who has health, has hope, and he who has hope, has everything.
—AN ARABIAN PROVERB

How to use this book?

Remember this is not a textbook on cardiology or a book which needs tremendous attention and background knowledge or technical knowledge. It is like a story. You don't need a highly scientific brain to understand the contents. It is for casual reading. Just note or underline the things which you need to follow. Re-read those underlined items later, with a little more attention, you may note them separately.

I have given a short introduction like many other books. This chapter will tell you the purpose of the book and a rough idea of the full contents.

Take a closer look at the contents again:

Many receive advice, only the wise profit by it.

— SYRUS

Contents of the book at a glance

You have already gone through the introduction. Here, I have tried to discuss the most commonly asked questions: "Is the reversal of heart disease possible?" "Is cardiology progressing?" and so on. I have also given a brief account of the SAAOL Heart Program.

The second section explains everything about the heart and the disease. What is the heart? How does it look? Why is it important? How does it get its blood supply? What is collateral circulation? This chapter also gives you an idea about the facts and figures of the incidence of heart disease in India.

The third section deals with the cause of heart disease and the risk factors. Each of the factors starting from cholesterol and triglycerides to stresses has been described in this chapter.

One must remember, this is what will form the basis of our treatment of SAAOL. I have also discussed things like — What is heart disease? How do deposits take place? Where do they occur? How to analyse the reasons or deposits? Just apply your mind, these questions will automatically come up. Even a child can apply his mind and ask these questions. As you go through the book you will know the answers. Ask yourself the questions and then read the answers. Everything is going to be clear.

The fourth section is about the tests being conducted on heart patients — to confirm the disease, the stage of the disease, to predict the prognosis and to follow the patient's improvements. You will learn about the tests like the ECG, Echo cardiogram, Stress test, Thallium test, Lipid profile test and so on.

I would advise this chapter to be read before you go on to the treatment chapters (i.e. Sections 7, 8, 9, 10, 11) so that you can understand every aspect and component of the SAAOL and other treatment systems.

The fifth section deals with the understanding of a heart attack, the state all heart patients are fearful about. Without this knowledge patients of heart disease would never get confidence in life. One must be convinced that if he or she knows what to do — heart attacks are completely avoidable. This chapter is, thus, very important for every heart patient or his close relatives.

The sixth section is the chapter to understand the ongoing allopathic treatment system, part of which I also use under the SAAOL Heart Program. In this chapter I have tried to explain the medicines used by cardiologists and surgical procedures like bypass. I have tried to explain why all these systems are going to fail ultimately. During the development of the SAAOL system I came across so much unnecessary opposition from these ongoing systems being practised widely that I may sometimes

> The pen is the tongue of the mind.
> — Don Quixote

have been a little crude or sarcastic, for which I apologize now. The bitterness sometimes gets expressed inadvertently!

The seventh section is about the history and rationality of the theory of reversing heart disease. Why and how life-style is the only answer? I have tried to justify all aspects of what I have seen in my patients who have done tremendously well with their heart disease. Reading about them, will give you an insight about the totality of the program.

The life-style treatment of a heart disease has four important components — stress reduction, diet, yoga and exercise. Each of them have been explained in the following sections respectively (Sections 8, 9, 10, 11).

The twelfth section contains very important charts, questionnaires, tables and forms, which will be very useful when you start following the program. Please use them for best results and keep a track of your follow-up and progress.

I have devoted the last few pages of the book to tell you about some of my patients, their comments, our additional activities and other miscellaneous information, which I thought would be useful. Some important addresses of our offices in other cities are also included in this section. This is the thirteenth section of the book.

Don't listen to anyone who tells you that you can't do this or that. That's nonsense! Make up your mind, then have a go at everything. But never, never let them persuade you that things are too difficult or impossible.

— Douglas Bader

Specific details of the book

This book is both a story of the heart disease and details of its remedy. It is not meant for a medical doctor or cardiologist who is going to appear for an examination. It is meant for people who do not understand complicated and technical medical terminology. I have purposefully tried to simplify or sometimes oversimplify medical terms so that the common man can comprehend them without sacrificing the scientific validity.

Of course, for a doctor, who wants to read the book as a lay person, this book will be an enjoyment, as he would understand everything immediately and also realise how effectively we have moulded hard-core scientific information for the benefit of patients.

However, for those few who are in the quest of more scientifically oriented statistical details about heart disease, I would be happy to recommend a detailed reading of medical textbooks and books meant for cardiologists. There is no end to information on heart disease, but trying to pass all that information to someone who cannot grasp even 1% of it would be foolish and would defeat the purpose.

This book gives all practical information and instructions to the readers so that they are able to maximally implement them in their life. I understand a very simple fact that coming from different educational backgrounds, with varying degrees of analytical minds, many people would not be able to understand or follow all the instructions given in this book. But the assurance is that whatever little they follow, the results will be there for that part of the follow-up. I would however like to tell them to continue seeing their own physician (not necessarily a cardiologist) at regular intervals to find out relevant changes in the medicines, if needed, once they improve.

Though this program has been effective in treating thousands of severe heart patients, one must remember that every human machine is a little different in structure and function. There may be exceptional cases that may not respond adequately and nobody can guarantee their treatment by this program. Exceptions are there in every field.

In the SAAOL Heart Program we strongly recommend a change in life-style to reverse heart disease but till the patient improves the prescribed allopathic medicines are to be simultaneously continued and are only to be changed or withdrawn after a qualified physician advises so. Please keep this in mind.

Lastly, reading this book and following the life-style advised would always be inferior to the practical training that we impart as part of the SAAOL Heart Program. I would advise the readers to try and join the program to obtain maximum benefit.

The groundwork of all happiness is health.

— LEIGH HUNT

Why five steps? The power of five

Heart disease is a multifactorial disease — which means it occurs because of a number of causes. Naturally, tackling one of these causes would not be an effective solution.

The SAAOL Heart Program, now popularly followed in every part of India, utilises five major steps to treat heart disease non-invasively. These steps are to be followed totally and very accurately. Of course, the design of the program is so practical that every person can follow it. Each of these five steps has components and all these sub-components have different roles to play in the reversal of heart disease. It is this overall completeness of the program that makes it so effective.

Let me explain it again. When we have five iron sticks separately, anyone of them can be bent. But by putting them together, the strength increases tremendously and it becomes impossible to bend them.

Think of our hand. If I have only one finger, say the index finger, I can do ten kinds of jobs with it. With another finger added, say the thumb, I can do hundreds of jobs. With all the five fingers together I can do thousands of jobs. The efficiency increases tremendously as soon as the whole hand is complete.

This exponential enhancement of power of the program, with additions of all the sub-components, makes it possible to get the results quickly and effectively.

These five steps are education, stress reduction, diet modification, yoga, meditation and exercise.

Education and explana-tions in the language that laymen can understand makes it possible for heart patients to know the details about the disease and the theory of reversal. Patients must know the optimum levels of blood pressure, blood glucose, cholesterol, triglycerides and the effects of all these on heart disease. The reasons for blockages, ways to study them, diagnosis and tests to study heart disease, effects of medicines and the types of medicines — all are to be understood by the patients.

The program instructs heart patients in detail as to how to follow stress reduction, behaviour change, complete dietary know-how, yoga practice, meditation and exercises for different degrees of heart disease. All the instructions are to be followed in totality. Please keep this in mind.

Only do always in health, what you have promised to do when you are sick.
— SIGISMUND

What you need to reverse heart disease is accuracy

Any work which is to be done successfully, needs accuracy. For reversing heart disease this is very important. Not that the lifestyle changes were not known before the development of the SAAOL Heart Program, but the problem was inaccuracy and lack of complete knowledge. Heart disease is caused by a number of reasons and to cure it, you need to know all of them in a precise manner and practically to implement the knowledge.

If things are not done in the exact manner the results will also be illusive. Accuracy can only be achieved by years of scientific research and efforts. Many people who are not trained in the medical aspects of the body and development of heart disease may also venture to become doctors promising heart disease reversal. This may prove to be dangerous.

The failure of preventive medicine or cardiology is mainly because it was taken lightly and because it was used mildly. Results did not follow the treatment. Many people or doctors who are advocating less accurate life-style to prevent or slow down the progress of heart diseases are also creating a wrong trend. Some have allowed little oil, fish or foods with high oil content in the diet, some have avoided the training of stress management (which is very important for reversal). Most people lack the completeness of the concept, diluting the treatment process, often at the cost of adequate results.

I have tried to give the maximum information about what can be done and followed. But it should not be compromised from any aspect. Please try to contact us in case you are not confident or need personalised advice.

For extreme diseases, extreme strictness of treatment is most efficacious.
— HIPPOCRATES

Know Your Heart and Disease

Contents

Introduction

Coronary heart disease (constitutes more than 95% of heart ailments) can be called the 'disease of ignorance', as it develops due to lack of knowledge. If proper knowledge is imbibed, it will be very rare for a person to develop heart disease. But this knowledge must not remain only in medical books, it must be disseminated to common people. Knowledge should be simplified so that it can be easily understood.

Half the solution lies in the knowledge about heart disease. The human body is one of the best machines in the world and if maintained properly it cannot develop a snag. Heart disease is actually a result of a long period of mis-management of the heart by following a wrong life-style. With wrong food, excess fats and cholesterol, uncontrolled diabetes and high blood pressure, low exercise, smoking and consumption of tobacco and excessive stress, people start developing blockages in their heart tubes. Starting is always from zero. With repetitions of the same, year after year, blockages increase till the person reaches the range of about 70%. And that's when heart disease is diagnosed.

> One gentleman came to me after he had a re-blockage, 2 years after a bypass surgery. I saw all the papers and saw the bypass surgeon's note. When I asked him how he had got the blockages again, he said, "I don't know." He was totally ignorant about the blockages or the causes. Everyday he was eating chicken and butter. Curious to check his knowledge about his operation I asked him, "What surgery did you have?" Promptly came the reply, "There was a bone growing in my heart and the doctor removed the growing bone." He opined, "Doctor I feel the bone has grown again."

> Both physicians and patients must come to terms with the inability of medicine to postpone death indefinitely.
>
> — J. BLACKHALL

While treating heart disease by life-style change, I realised that many people were not aware of what was actually wrong with them or their heart, though they had been taking medicines for years or had even undergone bypass surgery.

When I started the treatment for reversal of heart disease, I found that the first thing the patient needed to know was about the heart machine — how it functions, how it looks, which are the arteries (tubes) that get blocked, why is there pain or choking, how much blockage is needed to create the symptoms. What is a heart attack? How does the blockage grow, what are the reasons for the growth of blockage, what is blood pressure, what is cholesterol, what is triglyceride and so on. Without knowing these, they never feel confident. I find that most of the doctors do not have the time or expertise to explain the same. In this chapter I am going to explain all this. Without knowing all this, it is virtually impossible to reverse heart disease.

One patient came to me with complaints of angina. When I enquired about his serum (blood) cholesterol, he proudly said, "I get it tested every year and I have no cholesterol." I asked him about the exact figure ? He did not remember, but I made him call up his home. It was 245 mg/100 ml., one of the highest that a heart patient can have! This is mis-information. The normal cholesterol level is 130 to 200 mg/100 ml.

One gentleman came to me with heart disease. He was overweight. When I told him that he was overweight by 20 kilograms he was unmoved. When I insisted, he said, "But sir, I have always been like this for the last 10 years." When I showed him the height-weight chart and explained to him how he was actually overweight, he said, "Doctor, actually my weight is okay but my height is less."

One more problem about educating heart patients is not about teaching — it is unlearning the wrong information. So much of wrong information has already gone into the patient's mind that it is almost impossible to rectify the mis-information.

No knowledge can be more satisfactory to a man than that of his own frame, its parts, their functions and actions.

— Jefferson

Coronary disease — different names

Whenever we talk about heart disease, remember we are mostly referring to the disease which is caused by the accumulation of fat and cholesterol in the arteries (blood carrying tubes in the walls of the heart). It accounts for more than 95% of the heart ailments. This means that out of 10 patients with heart ailments more than nine will have obstruction in the blood flow to the muscles of the heart.

This disease of blockage of the heart arteries is medically called 'coronary heart disease (CHD)'. Over the years the same disease has been referred to by different names. The most common of these names is 'angina'. Angina means a pain on the left side of the chest often radiating to the left arm. Since this pain is commonly found in 80% of the people having coronary heart disease, angina also became a common name.

It is known that many patients of CHD do not have a typical chest pain but have shoulder pain, breathlessness, choking sensation or burning sensation in the middle of the chest. These are also due to blockage. So, we must know that CHD can occur without angina pain.

A little less known name of the same disease is 'ischaemia'— (shortage of oxygen). All the problems of the CHD occur due to shortage of oxygen (of course due to the blockage in the tubes supplying blood to the heart muscles). 'Ischaemia' is a more scientific term. CHD is also referred to as the ischaemic heart disease or IHD, and is still being used by many doctors and patients.

Another name of the disease is coronary artery disease (CAD), which is a more appropriate name and is now gaining popularity with doctors and cardiologists.

Of all the ailments which may blow out life's little candle, heart disease is the chief.
— WILLIAM BOYD

Stories about angina

Patient – A

Mr. S Lal, 47, a busy executive staying in Delhi had not suffered from ill health for a long time, and had never taken medicine. A few months back, he felt a heaviness of on the left side of the chest. He felt it while climbing the stairs. He ignored it, thinking it may be due to tiredness. But within a month the heaviness was replaced by a pain in the left side of the chest. He found it was radiating to the left arm. Just to check whether it was due to lack of fitness, Mr. Lal started going for a morning walk. As soon as he would walk about 500 yards, the pain would appear again and it would go off after he stopped and rested. He told his wife about it. Next day they were with their family physician, Dr. Puri, narrating the story. The ECG taken did not show any change. Dr. Puri referred him for a further test called the 'Stress Test' or 'Tread Mill Test'. The test was positive after 3 minutes on the machine. Mr. Lal was told that he suffered from angina or Coronary Heart Disease.

Later, Mr. Lal was told that his smoking habit, high cholesterol and excessive stress were the real causes of his pain and coronary blockage.

Patient – B

Mr. Ashok Patel, 42, had always been an overweight businessman in Mumbai, having a long standing diabetes or high blood sugar. He was taking some tablets and was getting a six monthly check-up of his blood sugar. Mostly the blood sugar figures were on the higher side. He was concerned but there were more pressing problems in the business, which he wanted to expand. He knew he should also reduce his weight. Lately he noticed that he got breathless while climbing the railway bridge on his way to work. Unknowingly he would slow down his pace and rest in the middle of the stairs. It was not like this earlier. He thought it was due to overweight. He thought of heart disease, because he knew being a diabetic patient, he had a higher risk of heart disease. But he assured himself that there was no chest pain. It could not be heart trouble.

He mentioned this to his business colleague in the shop, who suggested he meet a MD physician. Mr. Patel was diagnosed to have heart disease the very next day with a test called the Computerised Stress Test. The blockages were more than 70%.

Patient – C

Mr. Krishnamurthy, a retired government servant in Bangalore, was feeling a burning sensation in the middle of his chest, especially after meals for the past one year. He was thin, careful about his food and exercise. But he had had a very tough working life throughout his career and stress was still a part of his life. He was the secretary of the residents' association of the colony and also involved himself in various other social activities.

He attributed this burning sensation to gastric problem. He would take a Digeine or Gelusil liquid after meals when the burning sensation was more apparent. He noticed that this would go off after about two hours of meals. A doctor in his colony, whom he talked to casually, prescribed him stronger Antacid tablets (Ranitidine).

One day, after a heavy meal at a dinner party, Mr.

Krishnamurthy's pain was severe enough to make him visit his physician the very next day. The ECG on the same day confirmed that he was suffering from heart disease.

Patient – D

Mrs. Chatterjee, a housewife in Calcutta, was a little plump and a tobacco chewer for more than 20 years. A nice lady, with a lot of responsibility, as the head of a big family, she had a lot of help from her daughter-in-law. Everyday she would also go for a walk with her executive husband. She had a regular routine.

After a break of 15 days in the morning walk, while her husband was away on a business trip, Mrs. Chatterjee went for a morning walk again. In the middle of the walk she felt a choking sensation in her throat. She could not keep pace with her husband. Thinking she was tired, she sat down to rest. The whole day was normal. The next day the choking sensation was there again during the morning walk and whenever she stopped the choking disappeared This became a regular feature.

Mr. Chatterjee took her to a doctor, who gave her a routine check-up. Her cholesterol and triglycerides were high and she had the habit of chewing tobacco. She was given some Sorbitrate tablets. Now she would keep a Sorbitrate below her tongue before taking a walk and the choking would vanish. Her husband was informed that she needed to take a Tread Mill Test.

Angina — how to recognise it?

These four patients are some of the typical examples of heart disease. When a patient complains of a pain in the chest extending towards the left arm, diagnosis is almost coronary blockages. Pain usually aggravates on exertion and is relieved by taking rest. It is more apparent after meals, especially after a heavy meal. Many patients complain of breathlessness on exertion but not of pain in the chest. Many of these patients have diabetes and are overweight. Palpitation is also a common complaint of a heart patient.

Burning sensation in the middle of the chest, choking sensation, uneasiness over the chest region, chest pain during excitement, sometimes shoulder pain, right sided pain and jaw pain are also indicators of heart disease.

No age group is exempted from angina. Occurrence of angina at a younger age is a recent trend — basic reason being the process of atherosclerosis (deposition of fats and triglycerides) in the arteries that supply blood to the heart. Angina is unlikely till the blockage is more than 70%. The period over which these blockages are formed depends on the life-style of a person. If many risk factors are present and stress is predominant, angina can occur even at the age of 25 years. Previously angina was seen only at the age of 50-60 but now many patients with angina are in the age group of 30-35.

Recognition of angina depends on the patient's knowledge about the disease and physical activity. If he performs heavy

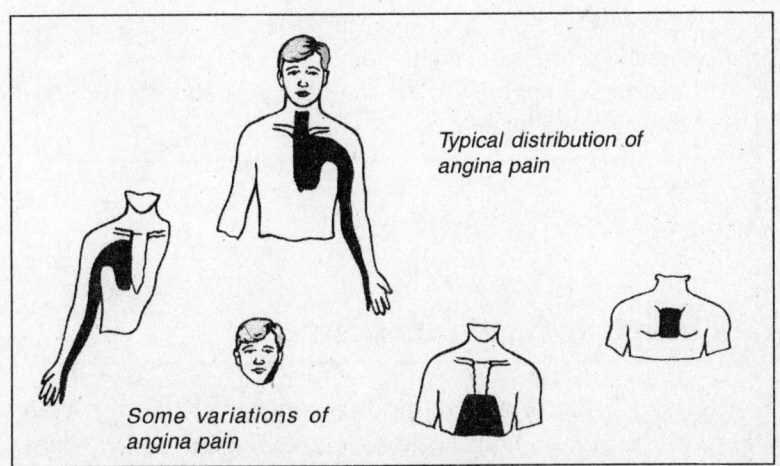

Typical distribution of angina pain

Some variations of angina pain

physical activity from time to time (where the heart rate is raised beyond 120-130/minute) he can identify angina early. People who do not physically exert themselves feel and recognize angina quite late, because they never reach a higher heart rate. Many such physically inactive persons sometimes get severe heart attacks which may even result in death, simply because they could not identify angina and take preventive care.

Angina does not occur at blockages of 40% to 50% which is widely prevalent. If it occurs, it is more likely to be precipitated by a sudden episode of coronary artery spasm which is the most common manifestation of stress.

The Symptoms of Angina

1. Chest pain: Angina may vary from mild to severe, whereas the pain of a heart attack is very severe. It usually occurs in the centre of the chest and radiates to the left arm, but at times it may even radiate to the right arm, shoulders or the lower jaw. The pain usually lasts for 5 to 10 minutes.
2. Breathlessness or shortness of breath.
3. Sweating.
4. Nausea and vomiting.
5. Dizziness and fainting.
6. Pain or heaviness in the chest especially after heavy meals.
7. Choking sensation in the throat.
8. Heaviness or tightness in the chest or upper abdomen.
9. Weakness and fatigue.

Fear always springs from ignorance.

— EMERSON

The heart and its functions

The human heart retains its priority among all the important organs of the human body because it is responsible for supplying blood to the entire human system, which is essential for the sustenance of our lives. Thus, it is of utmost importance that we should make every effort to familiarize ourselves with the heart and its functions.

The human heart is a small muscular organ situated in the centre of the chest, a little to the left. In size, it is roughly the size of a clenched fist and weighs about 350 gms. Since it is such an important and delicate organ, it is protected by the chest bone (sternum) in front.

Internally, the heart is divided into 4 chambers, and has four major valves. The upper two chambers are called the atria and the lower two, the ventricles. The right atrium receives impure or deoxygenated blood (blood which has been deprived of its oxygen content by the tissues) via veins from the entire body. This blood goes to the right ventricle which contracts and pumps it through the pulmonary arteries (blood vessels) connecting the heart to the lungs where it is oxygenated. The oxygenated or purified blood from the lungs goes to the left atrium via the pulmonary veins (the only veins in the human body to carry oxygenated blood) and into the left ventricle which contracts and pumps it with tremendous force throughout the body and supplies it to billions of tissues which make up the human body. This is how blood circulates in the human body.

As the heart is continuously working, it also requires oxygen and nutrition which is transported by the blood. Hence, the heart has its own blood supply. Blood is supplied to the heart through vessels called coronary arteries. There are two coronary arteries, the right and the left. The left coronary artery further branches into the left anterior descending coronary artery (LAD) which descends down in front of the heart, and the left circumflex coronary artery (LCx) which encircles the heart from behind. The right coronary artery (RCA) supplies blood to the front and back of the right side of the heart. All these coronary arteries have connections between themselves. We shall discuss about these arteries (tubes) that supply blood to the heart in a more detailed manner at a later stage.

.The heart is mostly made up of a strong muscle tissue called myocardium which works continuously like a tireless pump, day and night, throughout a man's lifetime. It beats about 72 times a minute, and if we calculate the number of minutes in our lifetime, it amounts to about 2.5 billion beats in a person's life-span of 70 years. It circulates about 7 litres of blood every minute, amounting to about 700 million litres of blood in a lifetime. During physical exercise and mental stress, this function can increase upto sixfold or even more; thus, making the heart the most efficient pump known to mankind. In spite of all the advances made in the field of science and medical technology, nobody has been able to artificially replicate such a pump.

The main function of the heart is to supply blood and essential nutrients to the whole body. Besides supplying blood, oxygen and nutrition to all parts of the body, the circulatory system also regulates the body's internal temperature, distributes hormones and removes the harmful by-products of metabolism, including a host of other functions which are beyond the scope of our discussion.

Functions of the heart

- Supplying blood to the entire body.
- Supplying oxygen and calorie nutrients (digested food particles that we eat) to the whole body and to billions of cells in the body.
- Supplying vitamins and minerals to cells of the body, without which they cannot survive.
- Carrying or pulling blood back to the heart and sending the

To know about your heart and its diseases

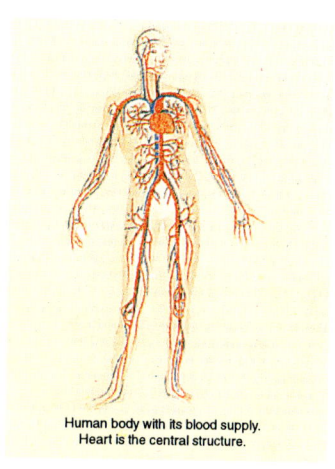

Human body with its blood supply.
Heart is the central structure.

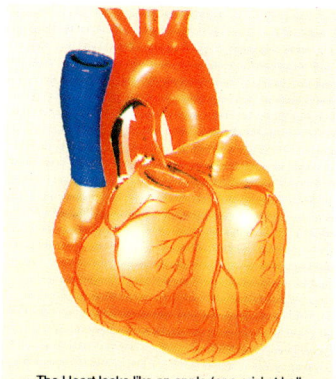

The Heart looks like an apple (or a cricket ball
which is hollow inside). The outer layer of muscle
(called Myocardium) gets supply from main artery
(Aorta) to the body through three coronary arteries.

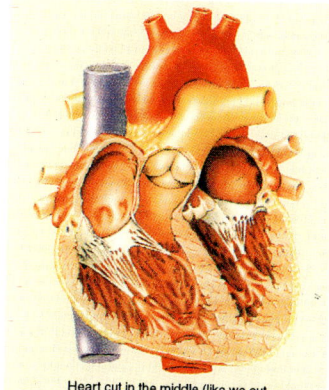

Heart cut in the middle (like we cut
an apple with a knife). You can see the walls
(Myocardium), the four chambers and the valves.

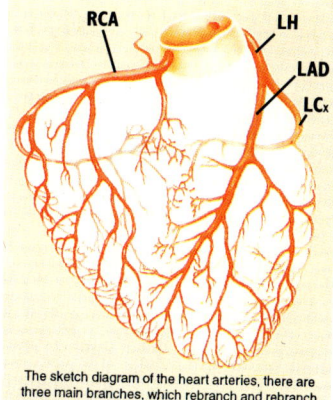

The sketch diagram of the heart arteries, there are
three main branches, which rebranch and rebranch
to supply the entire heart.

To know about your heart and its diseases

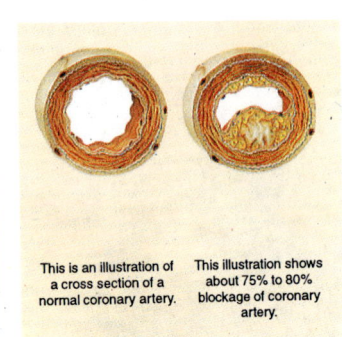

This is an illustration of a cross section of a normal coronary artery.

This illustration shows about 75% to 80% blockage of coronary artery.

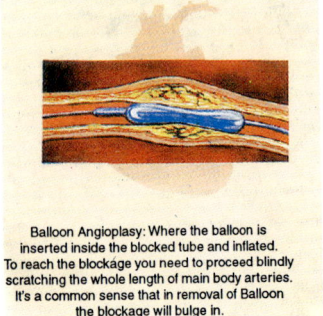

Balloon Angioplasy: Where the balloon is inserted inside the blocked tube and inflated. To reach the blockage you need to proceed blindly scratching the whole length of main body arteries. It's a common sense that in removal of Balloon the blockage will bulge in.

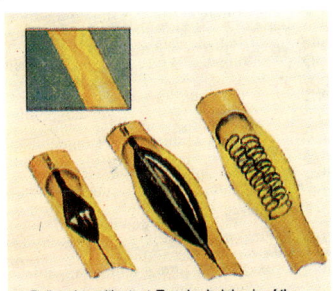
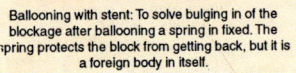

Ballooning with stent: To solve bulging in of the blockage after ballooning a spring in fixed. The spring protects the block from getting back, but it is a foreign body in itself.

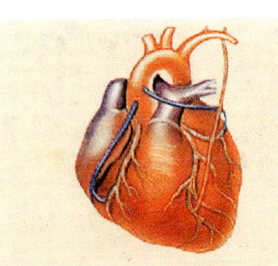

Bypass Surgery: A huge operation with so many complications costing a huge amount. The artificial tubes get blocked soon as the original did. Here two veins and one artery are used as graft the destiny is sealed in absence of life-style change.

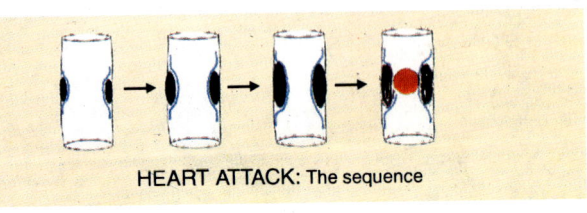

HEART ATTACK: The sequence

same to the lungs for a refill of oxygen.

- Help in distribution of hormones, neuro chemicals from one part of the body to another.
- Help taking the waste materials to the kidneys for purification of the blood. (The kidneys extract waste from the blood).

How does the heart pump the blood?

The heart has four chambers in a series, which pump the blood collected from the body to the lungs and then receive the purified blood (filled with oxygen) from the lungs and again pump the same to the whole body. These chambers are called right atrium (RA), right ventricle (RV), left atrium (LA) and left ventricle (LV). For a better understanding let's call them chambers 1, 2, 3 and 4.

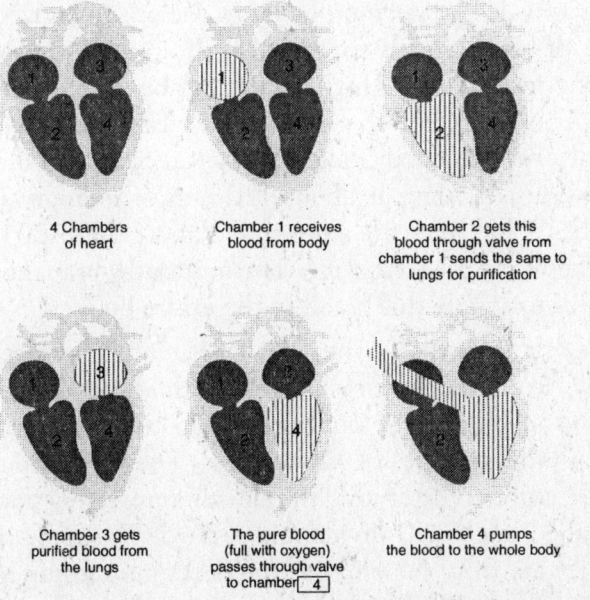

4 Chambers
of heart

Chamber 1 receives
blood from body

Chamber 2 gets this
blood through valve from
chamber 1 sends the same to
lungs for purification

Chamber 3 gets
purified blood from
the lungs

The pure blood
(full with oxygen)
passes through valve
to chamber 4

Chamber 4 pumps
the blood to the whole body

'Chamber 1' gets about 70 millilitres of blood almost every second from the entire body through two major veins (tubes carrying blood to the heart). This blood accumulates and is passed on to 'chamber 2' through a valve which opens only in one direction allowing the collected blood to pass in that direction. 'Chamber 2' contracts, thereby closing the valve between the first and second chambers, but opening another valve which pushes 70 ml. blood to both the lungs.

The blood now reaches the lungs for purification i.e. removal of carbon dioxide and filling up with oxygen. The lungs collect oxygen from the air that we breathe in through the nose.

Once the blood is purified it is sent to 'chamber 3' through some tubes and accumulates there. Then this blood is pushed to 'chamber 4' through another valve which only opens in the direction of 'chamber 4'. No sooner the blood reaches 'chamber 4' this valve closes.

'Chamber 4' is the strongest and the most useful chamber of the heart as it has to pump blood to the entire body. Once the 70 ml. of blood comes to 'chamber 4', it contracts vigorously resulting in building a high pressure (above 120 mm of mercury). This opens another valve and pushes the blood to the main artery of the body called the aorta. Since the blood pressure inside the aorta is about 120 mm of mercury (mmHg), 'chamber 4' has to create a pressure of more than 120 mmHg to push the blood into this tube. The aorta now branches and re-branches to supply this blood to the entire body.

The first branch that the aorta gives blood goes to the heart, Usually two branches are available to the heart — one on the right and another on the left to supply blood to the heart muscles, especially the muscles of 'chamber 4'. These two branches — the right coronary artery and the left coronary artery (more popularly called left main) divide and redivide to supply the blood that they get from the aorta to the heart muscles. Immediately after its origin, the left main divides into two branches called left anterior descending (LAD) and left circumflex (LCx) to supply to the left part of the heart.

> The condition of the heart is like that of a cashier in the bank. The cashier handles crores (one crore is equal to 10 million) of money everyday, but he cannot use it for himself or for his personal requirements. He has to depend on his own salary which forms a small part of the cash that he is handling. Likewise the heart also handles so much blood everyday through its chambers but can utilise only a fraction of it for its own use.

One must remember that once all the chambers of the heart contract a round, 70 ml. of blood is pushed. Since the heart chambers contract 72 times in a minute, a total of about 5000 ml. of blood is pushed to the whole body in 72 instalments.

The aorta, supplying blood, first circulates the blood to the entire body. It immediately gives a branch on the right side to supply blood to the whole of the right hand. The next branches are to the brain and left hand. It takes a turn below, and gives a series of branches, called arteries to the chest walls. Once it enters the abdomen it supplies blood to the liver, kidneys, spleen and intestines (both large and small). Finally it divides into two branches to supply blood to the legs.

Some simple but interesting facts about the heart

1. The heart beats about 72 times in a minute, about 4200 times in an hour and about 1,00,000 times in a day.
2. The heart needs about 250 ml. of blood in a minute for its own use.
3. The heart mainly utilises oxygen for converting food into

energy. But in an emergency it can break food particles without oxygen (anaerobic oxidation) for sometime.

4. The heart is an extraordinary device for maintaining blood circulation (slightly more than a gallon in the adult body) through approximately 60,000 miles of blood vessels.

5. Our body has about 5 litres of blood, and about 25 trillion red blood cells which carry oxygen from the lungs to all the body tissues. Everyday about 200 billion new red blood cells are released into the bloodstream and the old cells are removed.

6. During an average human life-span of 70 years, the heart pumps between 30-40 million gallons of blood. It beats nearly 2.5 billion times. Despite all the work it does, the heart is only the size of our fist. Despite its small size, the heart uses about 20 per cent of the total blood circulated to supply to its own muscles with oxygen. Unlike other muscles of the body, the heart works unceasingly, even while a person is asleep.

7. The heart is truly a remarkable piece of natural engineering. Day and night, whether we are sleeping or exercising, mere 250-350g of heart muscles continue to act as our vital pump, maintaining the circulation of blood through our body with a smoothness and coordination that any mechanical engineer could only marvel at, and certainly never hope to replicate it in a man-made system.

The tubes which get blocked — the coronary arteries

When the heart supplies the blood to the aorta (the main artery of the body) it retains two branches for its own supply. The muscles of the heart which have to contract continuously, need a continuous supply of blood. This blood brings food and oxygen — which gives it power in the form of calories.

The tubes are called coronary tubes, because when they divide and redivide, they look like a king's crown. There are two main tubes that form this crown. The one on the right side is called the right coronary artery or RCA, which has a diameter of 5 mm. It has a series of branches as it goes down and circles around the right side of the heart and proceeds as the PDA. This tube can be divided into three parts — proximal third, middle third and distal third.

The branch on the left is called the left main (LM) which immediately divides into two branches.

The first branch, the left anterior descending (LAD), is so named as it supplies to the front (called anterior in medical language) of the heart and goes down (called descending in medical language), supplies blood through numerous branches to the heart muscles. It supplies

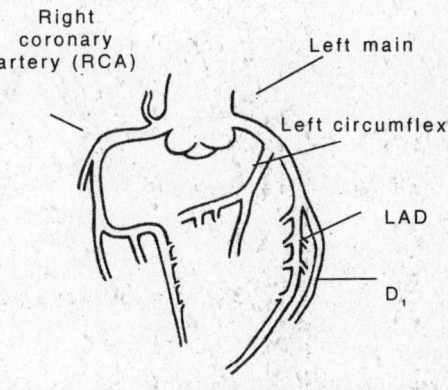

blood to some branches in the right, called the septal branches (named as S_1, S_2, S_3 and so on) and some in the left called diagonal branches (D_1, D_2, D_3 and so on). For purpose of easy description, this artery (LAD) can also be divided into three parts — proximal third, middle third and distal third. The LAD is bigger than RCA in size and is more important as it supplies to the main part of the heart 'chamber 4 or the left ventricle'.

The second branch on the left side of the heart is called the left circumflex (LCx) as it circles down the circumference of the heart on the left side. It is a little smaller than the RCA in size. The circumflex artery branches out to supply all the areas in the back of the left side of the heart. Some of the branches of this tube are called obtuse marginals and are expressed as OM_1, OM_2, OM_3 and so on.

The size of these branches varies from one person to another and there are often minute variations in the branches and supply areas. Seen from angiography (photograph of the heart after injecting radio-opaque dye) the branches look like the following diagram when seen from different angles.

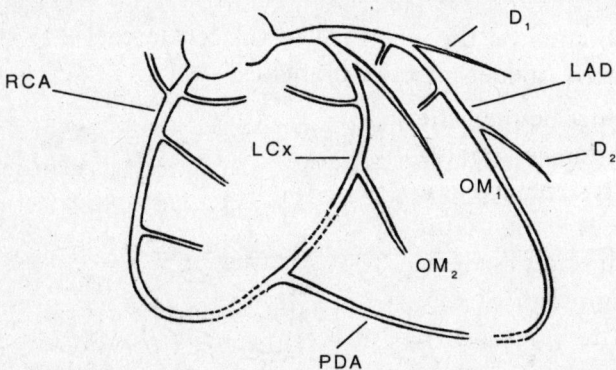

Diagram of the heart's blood supply.

How much blood does the heart get and need?

The heart is actually a pampered organ so far as the blood supply is concerned. It has provisions for blood supply of more than three times than it maximally requires. The tubes or arteries supplying blood to the heart are so big, compared to the size of the heart, that with even 70% blockage of the tubes the heart can still get adequate blood supply. Thirty per cent of open tube is good enough to ensure that even at the highest speed of running there will be no dearth of blood to the heart muscles.

When the coronary heart disease patients lead a wrong life-style it results in deposition of fatty substances, which lead to reduction in supply of blood to the heart muscles. Those who lead a reasonably healthy life-style may also have blockages upto 30% to 40% but will never come to know the deficiencies. Only those who consume wrong and excessive food and lead a very sedentary life and have a high level of stress can develop 70% blockage. This used to take about 30-40 years of reasonably wrong life-style to get a heart disease a few decades back.

But today, with the worsening life-style and no guidance from the health providers, this 70% blockage takes about 10-15 years. The destruction or closure work of the heart arteries proceeds at a greater speed. As a result we now see many young heart patients in 30-35 years of age.

Collateral circulation of the heart

The heart, as you know, is the best machine ever manufactured. In addition to the normal blood supply the heart has many dormant arteries, which can take over the functions once the normal arteries of the heart get clogged. These are called collateral arteries. They form a meshwork and can also supply blood to the adjacent arteries if an emergency arises.

When the heart functions normally even 30% of the existing arteries are good enough to supply blood to the heart, even at the peak of physical exertion. But in case the blood supply is reduced further (due to increased blockages) these collaterals take over. The collaterals are well developed in people who are physically very active and who have taken to sports.

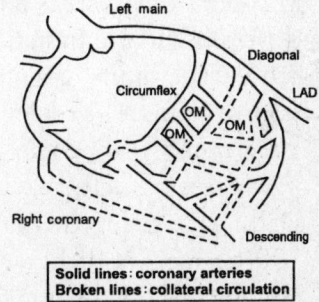

Collaterals can save many patients when they get a hear attack (100% blockage of a tube). This is often referred to as a 'natural bypass'.

Coronary Heart Disease: facts and figures in india

Heart disease is the largest killer in developed countries and is rapidly assuming a similar role in developing countries too. India too is undergoing an epidemiological transition and is on the threshold of an epidemic of cardiovascular disease (CVD). It has been predicted that CVD will be the most major cause of mortality in India by the year 2015. Demographic projections suggest a major increase in cardiovascular disease mortality due to increased life expectancy and life-style changes that are non-conclusive to CVD.

CHD has been rightly called the 'plague of the nineties'. Once believed to be a disease of the rich, prevalent mostly in developed countries, it is now striking Indians at an alarming rate. Recent studies have shown a high prevalence of CHD in both urban and rural population of India. In urban areas, it is as common as in the developed countries. Studies have shown a rising trend. Studies from rural areas have shown a lower prevalence as compared to cities but a rising trend is seen there as well. Surveys in Delhi's urban areas have brought forth a disturbing aspect of the disease in the Indian context. It expresses itself in the 3rd or 4th decade of life, engulfing a major percentage of our population. It is more prevalent among the younger population as a large number of people in their 30s and 40s are affected. Two new cases of CHD are being detected every hour in Delhi. If Delhi were to represent what is happening in urban India, then 100 new cases of heart disease increase every hour, which amounts to roughly 2500 cases each day.

Demographic Trends and Projections in India, 1981-2021

Population (millions)	1981	1991	2001	2011	2021
Total	683.2	844.3	993.7	1122.9	1253.8
%>35 yrs	28.4	28.8	31.9	37.1	42.4
Urbanization (% population)	23.3	25.7	32.1	37.9	42.8

Estimated and Projected Mortality Rates (per 100,000) by Sex for Major Causes of Death in India, 1985, 2000 and 2015.

	1985		2000		2015	
	M	F	M	F	M	F
Circulatory	145	126	253	204	295	239
All causes	1158	1165	879	790	846	745
Infections	478	476	215	239	152	175
Cancer	43	51	88	74	108	91
Pregnancy	0	22	0	12	0	10
Pre-natal	168	132	60	48	40	30
Injury	85	65	82	28	84	29
Others	239	293	180	185	167	17

Conservative estimates suggest that in 1990, CVD caused 2.386 million deaths and the nation incurred a loss of 28.592 million disability adjusted life years (DALYs). A two-fold increase of mortality attributable to circulatory factors between 1985 and 2015 has been predicted in the light of anticipated population growth and age structure. If the expected rise in urbanization and the rise in risk factor levels in the population accompanying altered life-styles are also taken into account, the rise in cardiovascular disease mortality is likely to be even higher.

CHD remains the leading contributor to global mortality and the epidemic threatens to attain a menacing magnitude as it advances and accelerates in the developing countries. The epidemic of CHD will be a public health disaster which will strain human as well as fiscal resources.

According to the American Heart Association, it is a fight that you can win. In fact, all it takes to turn these statistics around and stack the odds in your favour are a few simple precautions. Measures that can reduce risk of heart disease and increase your chances of a longer, healthier life. Therefore, the need of the hour is to develop cost effective preventive strategy with reference to tobacco control, promotion of physical activity, and reduction of stress using indigenous techniques like yoga and meditation and dietary modifications.

Consider some of these observations. Atherosclerosis (blockages) is largely a disease of technologically developed countries and recently of the developing countries also. Many human populations show a low incidence of cardiovascular disease, especially preliterate societies such as the tribes in New Guinea, Kung tribes in Kalahari Desert, and Eskimos in Canada and Greenland. Most mammals other than humans do not develop atherosclerosis. Animals in the wild are usually free from the disease — but some animals in captivity do develop atherosclerosis. These observations suggest that cardiovascular disease is not inevitable and that a particular style of modern living (stress, overeating, lack of exercise and smoking) is the real cause of high incidences of heart disease in this country or in the world.

References

American Heart Association Pamphlets.

CHD — Plague of the Nineties, *The Hindustan Times*, July 1914.

Gupta, Rajeev, et al: Prevalence of CHD and Coronary Risk Factors in an Urban Population of Rajasthan, IHJ, 1995.

Reddy, K.S.: *Cardiovascular Diseases in India*, World Health Statistics Q. 1993.

Reddy, K.S.: *Cardiovascular Diseases Control in India*, Cardio update, 1996.

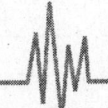

What Leads to Heart Disease?

Contents

Introduction

Coronary heart disease (CHD) or coronary artery disease (CAD) or ischaemic heart disease (IHD) is one of the leading causes of morbidity and mortality throughout the world. It is on a constant rise now in India too. The main cause of this disease is deposition of cholesterol and fat in the inner smooth lining of the blood vessels (coronary arteries) supplying blood to the heart resulting in their blockages and obstruction of blood flow through them. An atheromatous plaque is formed which compromises the flow of blood, oxygen and nutrients to the heart.

With significant blockages, more than 60% to 70%, and exertion, the increased demand of blood by the heart is not met, and a sensation of pain is felt in the chest which may also move down the left arm, typically called angina. This is a very dreaded condition and if left unattended may give rise to life threatening consequences.

Certain conditions and life-style habits are now recognized and documented to be responsible for the deposition of cholesterol and fat in blood vessels as well as the increased rate at which they are being deposited. Some of these risk factors have been mentioned below.

Risk Factors of Heart Disease

> All science is concerned with the relationship of cause and effect. Each scientific discovery increases man's ability to predict the consequences of his actions. And thus his ability to control future events....
> — LAURENCE J. PETER

Risk factors are the reasons which lead to or aggravate the deposition of cholesterol or fat in the coronary arteries. If one desires to know the total

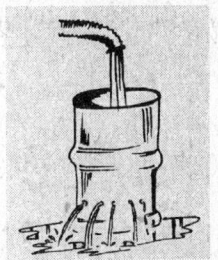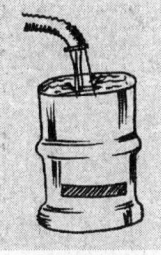

When there are twelve holes in a bucket — we have to close all the wholes to fill it up. The same applies to the treatment of heart disease where to control the disease one needs to control all the risk factors.

number of risk factors responsible for the development of coronary heart disease it will amount to hundreds.

Williams in 1981 identified 246 risk factors that directly or indirectly lead to the development and onset of heart disease. To give you a rough idea, the distribution of these risk factors is mentioned below:

Habits and lifestyle, psychosocial	54
Physical and biochemical	16
Serum / blood measurements	44
Medical conditions or diseases	45
Dietary deficiency (inverse association)	23
Dietary excess (negative association)	21
Constitutional, demographic	16
Blood clotting (platelet) disorders	16
Environmental	5
Drugs	6

If you consider the major 10 or 15 risk factors, those which are important in the development of coronary heart disease, they have been classified into two categories:

1) *Modifiable Risk Factors:* These include risk factors which can be altered and prevented so that further progress of heart disease can be arrested.

2) *Non-Modifiable Risk Factors:* These are risk factors which cannot be altered such as age, sex and heredity.

Modifiable Risk Factors

1. Stress and mental tension
2. High blood cholesterol
3. High blood triglycerides
4. Low blood HDL level
5. Lack of antioxidants in the diet
6. High blood pressure
7. Diabetes mellitus
8. Obesity or overweight
9. Sedentary life-style/lack of physical activity
10. Smoking or tobacco consumption

Non-Modifiable Risk Factors

1. Age
2. Sex
3. Heredity

Modifiable Risk Factors

Some of the above mentioned risk factors are described in brief.

Stress and mental tension

Psychological stress or tension is now recognized as the most important risk factor of coronary heart disease. With more and more scientific research results pouring in over the last 2 decades we have come to know that excessive stress can lead to the following:

1. Increase in blood pressure.

2. Increase in the heart rate.
3. Increased concentration of fat in blood.
4. Increased blood sugar.
5. Increased cholesterol in blood.
6. Spasm of coronary and other arteries.
7. Increased blood clotting.
8. Increased deposition of fat and cholesterol in the arteries.

This means that stress is such an influential risk factor that even in the absence of other risk factors it can by itself become responsible for coronary heart disease. I have seen many people without high cholesterol, overweight and family history, having normal blood pressure developing angina only because of excessive stress.

The problem with stress is that there are no means of measuring it even with the latest scientific gadgets. There is no unit, such as ml, mm, kg, etc., to define it. Because of this reason modern science and cardiologists have specifically abstained from talking about stress in heart disease. It is now known that city dwellers have 3 times more chances of getting heart disease than those in small villages, the major reason being excessive stress in city life.

Research has also revealed that a particular type of people (Type-A behaviour) who are aggressive, always short of time, short-tempered and stressful are much more prone to develop heart disease. Most young heart patients of modern day have Type-A behaviour.

It is obvious that without controlling stress we cannot stop the advancement of heart disease. Sudden stress or anger leads to the spasm of coronary arteries which precipitates sudden angina and heart attacks. This is the reason why many people

The power of the waterfall is nothing but a lot of drops working together.

develop heart attack when they are excessively strained or hear bad news.

High blood cholesterol

High blood cholesterol is one of the most known risk factors of coronary heart disease. Previously cholesterol was supposed to be the most important cause of heart artery blockages but with more and more research data coming in, it has become one of the first three risk factors.

Cholesterol is a type of fat particle present in the blood in small quantities. This waxy particle is made up of a single chain of fatty acid with 27 carbon atoms. The structure is so complex that this fatty acid is rotated in four rings — in combination called cyclo-pentano-perhydro-phenantherene ring. It is one of the most decorated molecules known to medical science. Cholesterol has very important functions in the body as it forms a part of the cell wall, nerve coverings and the brain cells. We cannot imagine life without this molecule. So important is the requirement of cholesterol in the body that the liver has a manufacturing capacity of the minimum amount of cholesterol required by the body.

But if this molecule is present in a high quantity in the body or blood, the excess can be deposited to create coronary blockages. Not only is the heart affected; high cholesterol can also get deposited inside the brain arteries, leg arteries and also in the skin below the eyes.

Cholesterol carried in the blood is in free form, which is very dangerous and it can be also carried in combination of proteins (known as lipo-proteins). There is a strong relationship of blood level of free cholesterol and the rate of deposition of blockages in the heart arteries.

> A man is never so happy as when his mind, his senses, and his heart are all working harmoniously together.
> — SENECA

Previously it was presumed

that a cholesterol level of 250mg/100ml of blood was normal and safe. This was about 20 years back. After further research, it was found that a level less than 220mg/100ml was okay in the next ten years. But the latest scientific research has now proved that any level more than 200mg/100ml is definitely not good. The normal range of this fat is now considered between 130 and 200mg/100ml of blood. The SAAOL Heart Program recommends a level of cholesterol lower than 160mg/100ml of blood to achieve optimum results.

Blood levels of cholesterol are high in those people whose diet is rich in cholesterol. Foods that contain high cholesterol are egg yolk, meat of any kind (mutton, beef, chicken, pork — both red meat and white meat, fish). Another rich source is milk and its products like ghee, cream, butter, ice cream, chocolates, paneer, curd etc. This becomes the culprit in vegetarians, who depend heavily on milk. Any other fat, especially the saturated fatty acids are used in the liver to manufacture cholesterol.

Cholesterol is mostly deposited in the heart arteries, after it is converted into LDL cholesterol, the so-called bad 'low density lipo-protein cholesterol'.

SAAOL recommends very low cholesterol (130-160mg/100ml) in the blood. The total intake of cholesterol in the diet of a person should be as low as 10mg/day. A chart containing the contents of cholesterol in most common foods is given in the diet section of the book. A vegetarian on milk diet consumes as high as 200-500mg cholesterol while a non-vegetarian consumes as high as 1000mg per day.

In most of the developed countries it is compulsory to put a display on the food labels — the exact content of cholesterol in every food. But unfortu-

> Like Bonnie and Clyde in their succession of stolen roadsters, triglycerides and cholesterol travel together on lab reports terrorising the American countryside.
> — HARVARD MEDICAL SCHOOL HEALTH LETTER

nately in India this is not done, and this makes it difficult for the general public to know what food to eat and what to avoid.

Regular physical exercise, stress management, stopping of smoking can also lead to lowering of the cholesterol in the blood, besides control of diet.

High blood triglycerides

The other fat, besides cholesterol, that has gained importance in recent research studies is triglycerides, a major cause of heart disease. Almost all the fats that we eat in our food are nothing but triglycerides. This is probably the other name for oils. Triglycerides also forms a part of the blockage.

Tri means three and glycerides comes from glycerol. Triglycerides is a combination of one glycerol molecule with three fats (or fatty acids). In other words, three chains of fat molecules (units) when attached to one glycerol can constitute triglycerides. These three chains of fatty acids, depending on the number of hydrogen atoms that they contain, can be saturated, mono-unsaturated or poly-unsaturated in hydrogen.

The understanding is pretty simple: if there are thirty slots for hydrogen in a fatty acid and all of them are filled up, it will be called saturated (with hydrogen) fatty acid. Most of the hydrogenated fats, like vanaspati, push hydrogen in high pressure into the fatty acid molecules to make the fat saturated. They take poly-unsaturated fat and before selling, convert them into saturated fat by adding hydrogen.

On the other hand, if one hydrogen is missing in the fatty acid chain it ceases to be saturated. Since it is unsaturated by one hydrogen only it is called mono-unsaturated fat. It is something like 29 hydrogen atoms instead of 30 (as in saturated fat). That makes very little difference.

> Cigarettes are the only legal products that when used as intended cause death.
> — LOUIS W. SULLIVAN, SECRETARY OF HEALTH AND HUMAN SERVICES

Thirdly, if more than one hydrogen is missing in the fatty acid chain (like 28 out of 30), this fat becomes poly-unsaturated. Literally and structurally there is hardly any difference between these three types of fats. They look alike as well. Even from the heart disease formation angle all of them contribute almost equally to the blockage formation. While one does 90% harm, the other two do 88% and 86% harm.

Almost all kinds of oil is 100% fat of any combination of these three kinds of fat. It is through the bad and unethical advertisements for promoting their products that the oil companies have created an impression that triglycerides is good for the heart disease (which is interpreted by the patients as 'helping to cure heart disease'). This is not a fact. I have given a chart of average content of oils for patients' use. Choose if you can.

The normal level of triglycerides in the blood is 60 to 160mg/100ml. SAAOL recommends less than 120 mg/100ml. More than 160 mg is associated with increased incidence of heart disease.

Small amounts of triglycerides are manufactured in the liver. All food items also contain some invisible oils also. These two combined can make up for the minimum amount of oil requirement of the body and SAAOL recommends no additional oil intake by heart patients.

Example

One doctor recommended 3-4 teaspoons of poly-unsaturated oil to a heart patient and told him, "It is good fat, you can have it." The patient immediately said, "Sir, if it is good, I shall try to have as much as possible. I want to be disease free as early as possible." The doctor said, "No, it is less harmful, that is why I am recommending it in small quantity." Patient replied, "Why do you have to prescribe harmful items?

> Hypertension is a disease of civilised life. Growing up in New Guinea or the northern forest of Brazil is a fine way to avoid the disease.
> —HARVARD MEDICAL SCHOOL HEALTH LETTER

If you say it is harmful I will not even touch it." The doctor was surprised, because most of his patients were happy with some harmful oil. In private practice the patients have to be kept happy as well and he had been allowing some harmful oil till now! Lesson: Catch the doctors.

Example

One gentleman after knowing that there are three kinds of triglycerides (saturated, mono-unsaturated, poly-unsaturated) visited a pathological lab for testing his lipid profile. Presuming that the poly type (poly-unsaturated) is good, he insisted at the pathological laboratory to find out the break-up of the triglycerides in his blood. The pathologist was amused and refused saying that the facility was not available. The patient said, "You should have this break-up. I want to increase my poly-unsaturated triglycerides in the blood. I am eating so much of these costly oils these days. Why can't you tell me whether it is really helping?"

Low HDL cholesterol

HDL cholesterol is the so called 'good' cholesterol and can be measured from a fasting blood sample. It has a very high affinity to bind cholesterol and can remove cholesterol from the blockages.

HDL cholesterol level in the blood should be maintained above 40 mg per 100 ml of blood to prevent heart disease. Indians are known to have low HDL cholesterol and it is often seen that the average HDL cholesterol in Indians is below 40 mg per 100 ml of blood.

High blood pressure

The normal blood pressure in adults is between 100/60 to 140/90 mm Hg. If the blood pressure is consistently more than 140/90 on two or more separate occasions, it is called high blood pres-

> Being overweight is like carrying suitcases throughout the day. Some carry small and some carry big ones. You cannot give it to any porter.
> — SAAOL

sure or hypertension. It is a very common disease and about 20% to 30% of adults suffer from hypertension all over the world, but a majority of the people are not even aware that they have this disease because it does not produce any symptoms in a vast number of cases. This is why this disease has been correctly called the 'silent killer'. High blood pressure puts an extra strain on the heart and the arteries supplying blood to the other organs of the body. Many diseases are caused by high blood pressure such as heart attacks, heart failure, kidney failure, stroke (damage to the brain), and damage to the eyes. Higher the blood pressure, greater are the chances of getting the above diseases, especially heart attack.

High blood pressure can be classified as mild, moderate and severe. It is also one of the major causes of deposition of cholesterol and fat in the coronary arteries. It damages the endothelial lining of the arteries, making them more prone to fat deposition. Besides a high intake of salt, psychological stresses are also implied as important causes of high blood pressure.

Diabetes mellitus

The normal levels of blood sugar in a fasting person are between 80-120 mg%. If the fasting level of blood sugar is more than 110 mg%, or after meals more than 160 mg%, it is called diabetes or high blood sugar. In diabetic patients, sugar can be detected in the urine also. Diabetic patients have a higher chance of developing coronary blockages. They are also prone to several other diseases like kidney damage, as well as damage to the nerves and eyes. Patients with diabetes are usually obese, have high blood pressure and high blood cholesterol levels, all responsible for blockages. Heart attacks may occur at a younger age in severe diabetics. The symptoms of diabetes are

> Cigarettes dull the facilities, stunt and retard the physical development, unsettle the mind and rob the persistent user of will power and ability to concentrate.
> — DICK MERRIWELL

increased thirst, increased urination and weight loss, but in some cases there may be no symptoms at all. It is important for heart patients to control diabetes. India has a very high number of diabetic patients.

Obesity or overweight

If the weight of a person is more than the upper limit of weight for that age and sex, he is called obese or a fat person. People who eat excess fat and do not do exercise put on weight. There are standard charts available from which one can find out whether one is overweight or obese. Obese individuals have greater chances of getting heart diseases. They have increased chances of having high blood pressure and diabetes and thereby blockages. Obesity can be prevented by eating low caloric food, avoiding fats, avoiding excess sugar, and doing physical exercise regularly. Fat people remain inactive and are also made fun of sometimes. Therefore, they tend to develop excessive mental tensions resulting in hypertension and heart attacks. The chances of getting a heart attack increases by 15 times for obese people as compared to lean and thin individuals. SAAOL recommends a slow but sustained reduction of weight for obese patients. A reduction of 2-3 kg. per month is ideal.

Sedentary life-style / lack of physical activity

Sedentary life or lack of exercise in our daily life has become the most important reason of heart disease in modern life. With modern technology, help from their wives, drivers, servants, peons, and staff, most of the executives have stopped doing any physical activity. Research studies have shown that low physical activity is often associated with high incidence of coronary heart disease. Regular exercise can break fat, decrease cholesterol, reduce blood sugar, control blood pressure, reduce

> A cigarette is some tobacco wrapped in a piece of paper having a fire on one end, and a fool on the other.

overweight by consuming stored fat in the body and make the heart more healthy and strong to respond well to unexpected physical activity needs. The absence of the same will have the opposite effect. Without exercise more and more people will be prone to heart disease, diabetes, high blood pressure, obesity and a low level of fitness. Besides, lack of physical activity may also lead to less flexibility, joint diseases, and so many other ailments.

Think of a typical person in a modern society. His life is literally sedentary. He gets up at 6 a.m., has bed tea, reads newspapers. These two sedentary activities will consume about two hours alongwith watching television. He will probably talk on the phone for sometime. And followed by a bath and a good breakfast. He goes to the office or shop by car, scooter or public transport, doing very low physical activity. Even if he plans to walk everyday, he mostly misses doing it.

In the office, he does a lot of writing, talking and computing — all requiring him to sit on a chair — the whole day. No exercise till now. Late in the evening he comes home in the car or by any other mechanical vehicle. He then sits and watches television, gossips, has a good dinner and goes to sleep.

No exercise at all throughout the day. Heart disease is bound to come one day, may be after 5 years. If one does not exert physically, one must cut down the fat intake or face the consequences.

It is seen daily that labourers, porters, farmers, athletes or people who go to office by cycle hardly have a heart disease. On the other hand, clerks, officers, executives, sedentary businessmen, lawyers, doctors, bankers are more prone to heart disease, because of lack of physical activity.

In the past people did not have these vehicles. They used to exert more — walking to the office, visiting other villages on foot, working in the fields, carrying their luggage themselves, grinding their grains, cleaning the house themselves. So they did not have heart disease as they would break all the fats and meats they were eating. Now things have changed, therefore the heart disease is coming closer.

Smoking or tobacco consumption

People who smoke (cigarettes or bidis in India) are four times (400%) more prone to develop heart disease as compared to the non-smokers. The Framingham heart study carried out in a small town of Framingham, USA, studied more than 5000 people and their families for more than three decades. It confirmed that smoking substantially increases the risk of heart attack. It was also shown in the follow-up studies of the same group, that even after cessation of smoking, people were still prone to heart attack. Researchers found that cigarette smokers, who quit smoking, are still more susceptible to heart disease even after five years.

Smoking induced risk for heart disease can be related to the degree of smoking and the risk increases with a longer duration of smoking. A person who smokes 10 cigarettes a day is almost at double the risk than one smoking 5 cigarettes per day.

Tobacco that is inhaled while smoking is the major cause of erosion of the inner lining of the coronary arteries. Out of the thousands of chemicals in tobacco — nicotine, tar, alkaloids etc. cause this damage and make the layer more susceptible to cholesterol and fat deposits. It is like painting the inner lining with glue which would catch cholesterol and stick it on the wall.

One must also remember that smoking is as bad as having tobacco in any form. *Zarda, tambaku, gutka, khaini*, snuffing, tobacco used to clean the teeth — popular in many parts of India — have equally bad results.

> To put alcohol in the human brain is like putting sand in the bearings of an engine.
> — THOMAS A. EDISON

Ideal height-weight for adults

Ht. in Cms.	Ht. in Inches	Average wt. for Men (in kilos)	Average wt. for Women (in kilos)
145	4'9"	-	46.0
148	4'10"	-	46.5
150	4'11"	-	47.0
152	5'	-	48.5
156	5'1.5"	-	49.5
158	5'2.2"	55.8	50.4
160	5'3"	57.6	51.3
162	5'3.8"	58.6	52.6
164	5'4.6"	59.6	54.0
166	5'5.4"	60.6	55.4
168	5'6.1	61.7	56.8
170	5'6.9"	63.5	58.1
172	5'7.7"	65.0	60.0
174	5'8.5"	66.5	61.3
176	5'10"	69.4	64.0
178	5'10.8"	71.0	65.3
182	5'11.6"	72.6	
184	6'4"	74.2	

Adopted from the Life Insurance Company of India

These also lead to blockages.

Smoking is bad for health as it causes damage to the lungs, resulting in bronchitis and asthma. It also causes lung cancer. Smoking can also aggravate the peptic ulcer and chewing tobacco can lead to gastritis. Staying in a big city has an effect of smoking 5-6 cigarettes. Those who live with smokers or work with them are now also prone to the bad effects of smoking.

They are also prone to develop heart disease. These people are called passive smokers.

Psychological stress and tension is also a known factor which leads to increased smoking, besides its addiction. Many people keep on shifting from one type of smoking to another, but this does not help. In many parts of India, like West Bengal, smoking is also considered a habit of the affluent and educated people.

Prevention of tobacco or smoking has to be taken on a war footing all over the world. It is astonishing that whereas tobacco smoking is reducing in the developed countries, in the developing countries it is increasing. The World Health Organisation (WHO) now has smoking prevention on its priority list.

Intake of alcohol

Alcohol intake is also a known risk factor of coronary heart disease — directly or indirectly. It has become associated with heart disease in many ways. Alcohol leads to increased triglycerides, owing to its similarity of structure with glycerol, a component of triglycerides. Many good laboratories do not take blood samples for lipid profile test (which includes triglycerides) if the patients have consumed alcohol in the last 12 hours.

Alcohol also adds huge calories to the patients. Many people eat a lot of fried items while drinking. This also adds to fat, cholesterol and calories. Alcohol is often associated with increased stress and bad interpersonal relationships in the family. Alcohol is also one of the major causes of liver disease and failure, besides gastritis and neurological damages.

> Life would be infinitely happier if we could only be born at the age of 80 and gradually approach 18.
> — MARK TWAIN

There has been some confusion about recommending of alcohol in some newspapers and medical journals. It has been shown that alcohol can increase the HDL levels in the blood, but it also increases the triglycerides — it does more harm than benefit to the patients. One must see all the effects rather than one isolated parameter.

Moreover, many of these research studies are carried out in countries where the temperature is very low and alcohol is used in quantities much more than what is consumed in India with its temperate climate. The extrapolations are not justified with regard to alcohol. Many studies have also shown that alcohol also leads to an increased incidence of heart disease.

Non-Modifiable Risk Factors

Age

Heart attacks are most frequent between the age of 40-55 years, but it is not unusual for heart attacks to occur even below the age of 40 years. These days we see an increasing number of heart patients at a young age. I have a few patients who have suffered a heart attack below the age of 25 years. Heart attacks occurring at younger ages are correlated to a strong family history of high blood pressure, diabetes and high blood cholesterol levels. Heavy smokers also get heart attacks below the age of 40.

Sex

Most of the heart patients are male though the number of females is on a steady rise. The incidence of heart attacks in females is markedly less before menopause as the hormone oestrogen protects them; the exact mechanism of this hormonal protection is yet to be clearly understood but after they attain menopause (by the age of 45 to 50), they are exposed to an equal risk of getting heart attacks as males. These days females are burdened with work and increased stresses both at home and at the workplace and have

> Mostly eating habits, not genetic factors, result in fat families.

thus become more prone to developing heart diseases.

Coronary heart disease can present itself in various ways rang-ing from mild chest discomfort to a heart attack or even sudden cardiac death. Once the disease sets in, whatever be its form, it relentlessly increases unless preventive methods are employed to check its course. Epidemiological studies on heart disease have shown a dangerous trend of the increasing incidence of coronary heart disease in India and other developing countries of the Third World. In accordance with the latest reports more than 13.7% of the adult population is suffering from coronary heart disease in India, and this figure is constantly on the rise year after year.

Heredity

Strong history of heart disease in the family makes a person predisposed to coronary problems in his life. This cannot be changed. But one must remember that food habits, exercise habits and stress pattern are the three main causes of heart dis-ease and are probably responsible for about 90 to 95% of the causes of heart disease.

Thus it is obvious that those who have a disadvantage from the heredity point of view should be more careful about their food habits, exercise, stress reduction and control of other coro-nary risk factors are concerned.

Most of the heredity effects among these persons come through excessive production of cholesterol and triglycerides in the liver. Liver makes these two elements little more than the body's requirement. Thus these people, even if they restrict their diet, may still have high cholesterol/triglycerides. Obviously, their chances of having a heart disease will multiply if they do not restrict the fat intake in food.

In many cases, even after strictly following the SAAOL Pro-gram, if these persons can still not control their cholesterol or triglycerides, I prescribe lipid lowering medicines to them as a last resort.

In nature there are neither rewards nor punishments; there are only consequences.

— ROBERT G. INGERSOLL

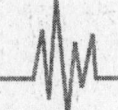

Diagnosis of Coronary Heart Disease

Contents

The fact that you don't know is enough of a curse; not to want to know is a fate that's much worse.

Introduction

Most of the patients suddenly have a panic reaction once they are told that they suffer from heart disease. Some who have more important priorities than illness, do not take it seriously and neglect the disease. In both cases, the cause remains ignorance about the gravity of the disease. This chapter explains the various tests performed on heart patients and their results. These tests include ECG, stress test (also known as TMT), stress thallium, echocardiography, Holter monitoring and so on. Knowledge about these tests would help the readers to know about the progress or reversal of the disease process also.

This chapter also explains about the meeting of patients with their doctors, the usefulness of detailed history taking and examination of the patients.

Though I do not prefer the angiography test, I am going to discuss this invasive test to highlight its faults and dangers and to disclose how it is used wrongly to put pressure on the patients to undertake bypass surgery or angioplasty.

Both physicians and patients must come to terms with the inability of medicine to postpone death indefinitely.

— Leslie J. Blackhall, MD

Meeting a doctor

Information/History Taking

The reliance on laboratory tests has increased as physicians attempt to utilise their time more effectively by delegating the responsibility of taking down the case history to nurses or assistants, who are not doctors or at times even by limiting the history to a questionnaire. This approach is undesirable as far as a patient with a known heart disease or suspected heart disease is concerned. It must be understood that the history remains the richest source of information concerning the patient's illness and any practice that might diminish the quality and quantity of information provided by the history is likely to impair the quality of care. Moreover the physician's attentive and thoughtful record of his patient's history establishes a bond with the patient that may be valuable later in securing the compliance of the patient in the future treatment plan.

Special History of Heart Patients

Whenever a doctor meets a patient with an expected heart ailment, the aim is first to confirm the symptoms related to angina. The typical pattern of pain in the left side of the chest radiating to the left arm almost confirms the diagnosis of angina (blockage of more than 70%). Mostly the pain is related to physical exertion and stops when the physical exertion is stopped. Some people complain about the aggravation of this pain due to emotional stress or after heavy meals. Many people complain of an uneasiness or suffocation or choking — which also suggests angina in 20-30% cases. Some diabetic people may not complain of chest pain but only of suffocation or breathlessness. This is basically because they don't feel the pain due to nerve damage because of diabetes.

The history of angina can also give an idea about its severity. Angina at rest is called Class IV angina. Class III angina means angina on slight exertion and Class II angina means that the patient can walk about 1-2 kms slowly without symptoms. Class I angina is a condition where the patient only gets a symptom after severe exertion like walking uphill, running or carrying weight.

In the case history, doctors should also enquire about past history of angina, heart ailment, high blood pressure, diabetes, smoking or tobacco consumption, family history of heart disease, food habits (vegetarian or non-vegetarian), past cholesterol reports and so on. All these reports not only lead the doctors to the cause of the disease but also help them to cure. They should form an important part of the patient's examination and often are more important than other advanced tests.

Unfortunately, most of the modern day cardiologists do not follow this practice. There are two reasons — one is the lack of time and second is that they are interested in getting either a surgery or angioplasty only and not in a long term improvement of the patient.

The most elegant of diagnoses is useless if the doctor cannot communicate its meaning to the patient or deal with the kinds of emotional response that interfere with the treatment of a disease.

— REBECCA A. JESSEE, MD

Examination of the patient

Examination is the second part of the doctor's duty after talking to the patient. The aim of the examination should be to look for risk factors like high blood pressure, checking of weight (overweight), swelling in the leg (pedal edema), pulse rate, and general examination. Listening to the heart sounds also gives a lot of additional information to the doctor about the state of the heart and they can also look for additional chest sounds.

Only after meeting and examining the patient, the doctor will know what investigations are required. He should then ask for an ECG (electrocardiogram) immediately to rule out any emergency if he suspects so. But in case he is sure that the patient is not in an emergency, he can proceed for the blood and other tests.

Blood tests for a heart patient

A. Serum Lipid Profile

This should be the first test to be recommended for a suspected or confirmed heart patient. This blood test should be done after 12 hours of fasting and gives the medical practitioner a fair assessment of the value of different fatty components present in the blood sample such as serum cholesterol, triglycerides, HDL (high density lipoproteins) cholesterol, LDL (low density lipoproteins) and VLDL (very low density lipoproteins). From this investigation the rate of deposition of cholesterol in the lining of the blood vessels or the breakdown of the deposits (reversal of blockages) can be predicted. The normal values of these tests are given in the table below. I always recommend people not to keep their value at the upper end of the range but to keep them at the lower end. For example, if the range of cholesterol is between 130 to 200 mg/dl — it is good to have a value which is closer to 130 mg/dl. This becomes more important for those who already have blockages in the heart arteries or those who have other risk factors which they cannot control due to circumstances.

Normal Range		
Cholesterol	:	130 to 200 mg/dl
Triglycerides	:	60 to 160 mg/dl
HDL (good) cholesterol	:	30 to 60 mg/dl
LDL (bad) cholesterol	:	50 to 120 mg/dl
VLDL cholesterol	:	12 to 35 mg/dl

Serum VLDL is usually estimated as one fifth of serum triglycerides.

Unfortunately enough, I have seen numerous heart patients being prescribed all sorts of blood tests in cardiology hospitals other than this most important blood test. Even angiographies and bypass surgeries are being done on these patients without even looking at the lipid profile.

It is a routine procedure to collect so many blood samples from heart patients and do tests like Australia antigen, AIDS sero tests, urea, creatinine, total and differential blood counts, urine tests and so on. Most of these tests are done in order to prepare the patients for procedures called bypass surgery or angioplasty.

Since heart disease is caused by fats, which exists in different forms in the bloodstream — heart patients are recommended to get a lipid profile test. This is a blood test where the parameters usually tested are — cholesterol, triglycerides, HDL cholesterol (good cholesterol), LDL cholesterol and VLDL cholesterol. Blood has to be collected after 12 hours of fasting in this test.

LDL Cholesterol = Cholesterol - HDL Cholesterol - 1/5th of Triglycerides

Blood glucose and glycosylated haemoglobin

Diabetes mellitus has a strong association with coronary heart disease and is responsible for the increased rate of deposition of cholesterol. Its control is a must. The level of glucose in the blood is monitored by periodical blood sample checks. For all the fasting samples blood should be collected after 12 hours of fasting and for the after food (called post prandial or simply PP) blood should be collected after 2 hours of a normal breakfast. The normal blood glucose level permitted to a heart patient is fasting 70 to 110 mg/dl and PP 120 to 150 mg/dl. However, I expect my patients to keep a fasting blood sugar below 100 mg/dl or lower, post prandial sample should be of course towards the lowest i.e 120 mg/dl.

Serum glycosylated haemoglobin (Hb A 1c) is another latest

and very important test for a diabetic patient and it should be done every two months. This test offers a gist of last two month's blood sugar control at one go. The results vary from 6% to 12% depending on the degree of blood sugar control. The lowest figure is the best.

ECG or electrocardiogram

ECG is the simplest and easily available test for a heart patient. This is an electrical recording of the heart. ECG reflects the proper functioning of the heart muscles and their condition as a function of the blood supply and oxygen received by them.

A single ECG curve has five main components — p, q, r, s, t. The space between s and t, called the ST segment can indicate angina, during the recording of the heart-beat. ST segment lowering (medical term is depression) is taken as a sure sign of angina. T wave inversion is also a sign of angina.

A doctor has to have a training of more than five years to be able to analyse the ECG. Even then it may be difficult for him to

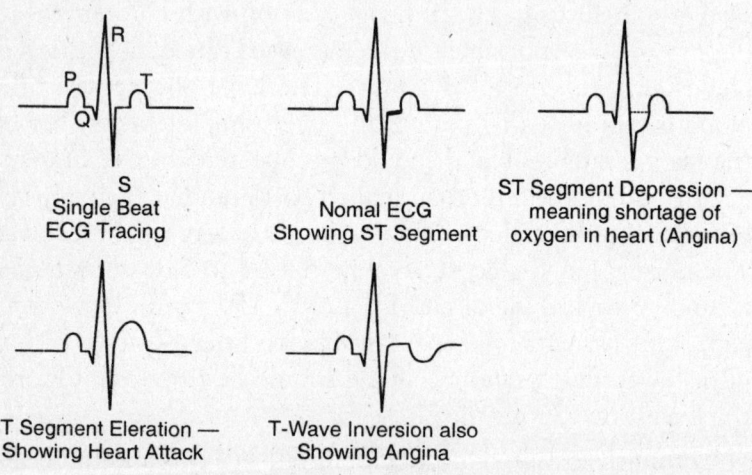

Single Beat
ECG Tracing

Nomal ECG
Showing ST Segment

ST Segment Depression —
meaning shortage of
oxygen in heart (Angina)

ST Segment Eleration —
Showing Heart Attack

T-Wave Inversion also
Showing Angina

know everything about it. It is advisable that the final decision should be taken only after the ECG is seen by a qualified doctor.

ECG is a simple and convenient investigation which can be done at the bedside to observe angina.

When breathlessness is felt, if ECG changes appear early in the TMT, then the coronary heart disease is severe, and if the changes appear later they are not so severe.

ECG was invented by Einthoven, the great scientist.

Echocardiogram

This is a non-invasive investigation based on the principle of interpretation of ultrasound used to assess the functioning of the heart muscles, their blood supply and the condition of the cardiac valves. It also gives us information regarding previous heart attacks and about the efficiency with which the heart is functioning.

During echocardiography the patient lies on the bed and the doctor puts a probe on his/her chest through which ultrasound waves are thrown to the heart. When these waves are reflected back from different parts of the heart — the same probe receives it and feeds the data to the computer. The computer after analysing the data can put the exact picture of the heart as a diagram. This diagram can supply information about the heart size, chamber size, valve defects etc — which is the outcome of the echocardiogram.

Echo can also give the pumping power of the heart (i.e. that of chamber 4 or the left ventricle). This is called left ventricular ejection fraction (LVEF). In a normal person the EF is 60% or so. This figure becomes lower after a heart attack depending on the severity of the heart attack.

Echocardiogram does not give any idea about the coronary blockages. Patients with multiple blockages can even have a normal echocardiogram report.

TMT or stress test

It is quite common to find heart patients who have a normal ECG. One must remember that the ECG is taken at rest when the heart is beating at its lowest rate. Even with 90% blocks the patient can have a normal ECG. In such a case the patient would also agree that at rest there is no pain in the chest, the angina symptoms would only come when the heart rate is increased while doing some physical exertion like walking.

This is when we need a TMT test. The patients are to gradually increase their heart rate, thus increasing the blood requirement of the heart muscles. Simultaneously ECG records are taken. If there is a blockage of approximately more than 70% ECG shows changes, which indicates angina.

Patients have to physically exert for this test which uses a computerised machine. The level of exercise is gradually increased according to a standard protocol called the Bruce's Protocol. The continuous ECG monitoring would reflect any blood and oxygen deficit in the heart muscles during exercise. The patient is asked to stop exercising as soon as ECG changes appear or any symptoms of chest pain or discomfort or breathlessness are felt.

TMT test is also called exercise stress test, computerised stress test or simply stress test. This is the most easy, popular and common test performed on heart patients to determine the severity of the heart disease. Taken at an interval, this test can also show the improvement or deterioration of the patient's angina.

A negative TMT or stress test is declared when the patient can reach a certain heart rate without showing any ECG changes.

This rate is called a target heart rate and is calculated by a formula (target heart rate = 220–patient's age). If this rate is reached by the patient without producing any ECG changes, though the TMT can be called negative, it would not necessarily mean that the blockage is zero. It will only mean that the person performing the test probably has a blockage less than 70%.

If at a pulse rate of 64 per minute the heart needs an oxygen supply of 267ml per minute, the heart will need about 300ml of oxygen per minute if the heart rate goes up to 173 beats per minute. This means that if the heart rate almost triples the oxygen requirement will go up by 11 times approximately. This also forms the basis of the exercise stress test or TMT.

PET scan

PET scan is the latest non-invasive investigation to ascertain coronary artery disease progress or the reversal of blockages. Dr. Dean Ornish used this investigation to show that reversal in the blockages of the coronary arteries of his patients had occurred. This extremely expensive and sophisticated investigation is available only in a few centres of the world. The patient is made to lie down on a table which is introduced into the scanner and sectional pictures are taken of the heart. A coloured graphic representation of the blood flow throughout the heart can also be obtained giving an accurate idea of the blockages present.

The PET scan machine costs around Rs.15 crores and is not as yet available in our country.

Thallium scan

This particular test study is done to assess the blood flow to the heart muscles during exercise (stress) or rest. A study can be made with the patient walking on a treadmill or even by infusing drugs, which increase the heart rate. Important precaution to be taken here is that if drugs are used to increase the heart rate then an asthmatic patient should stop taking Theophylline or Aminophylline 36 to 48 hours prior to the test.

It takes about 3-4 hours to complete the test. At the beginning of the test, the patient is placed on the treadmill, bicycle or is infused with drugs. The heart rate is allowed to increase until projected rate is achieved (or 4 muscles period after drug infusion). Then, Thallium-201 is injected and allowed to circulate for approximately 15 minutes, while the patient maintains the projected heart rate. The patient is then placed under a nuclear camera and images are recorded which show how the Radioisotope has circulated to the myocardium. The patient is asked to return for another set of pictures taken at rest 2-4 hours later.

After this the physician compares the heart at rest as well as under stress. Areas of the heart muscles which show a good uptake of Thallium-201 means the arteries are open and on the other hand the heart muscles which show no uptake of Thallium-201 are considered to have impaired blood flow and means that there is a blockage in the coronary artery supplying blood to that area of the heart.

Stress muga

This is yet another non-invasive test and quite similar to stress thallium. The particular purpose of this test is to measure and assess the ejection fraction of the left ventricle (chamber 3 of the heart). In stress muga the patient is given two injections, the first one is a non- radioactive drug and is followed by a second injection, approximately 20 minutes later, of a very small amount of radioactive tracer. The patient is then placed under a nuclear camera and the images of the heart are taken. This can be performed with or without exercise. The normal ejection fraction ranges from 60-66%.

Helical CT angiography

The aim of this type of angiography is to visualise the lumen of an artery by non-invasive techniques.

In this process a contrast is given to the patient in a peripheral vein with an electronic pressure injection syringe about 100-150 ml of contrast and an appropriate scan delay is employed to ensure that the contrast reaches the target organ. A spiral sequence is then acquired within a few seconds and thus the patient is out in less than 5 minutes.

Once helical data has been acquired, the images are reconstructed and analysed along with multiple post processing techniques. What is now gaining prominence is the CT angioscopy, whereby one can have a view of the vessels from inside, thereby commenting on the blockages of the vessels (still in process).

CT angiography is suitable for almost any part of the body, but the ones that are normally done are the arteries of brain, neck, arms, abdomen, kidney and lungs. Recently they have visualised the beginning of the coronary arteries. Probably soon they will be able to do a four dimension CT and will be able to see the three dimensional picture of the heart, pulsating in real time with the blood flow visible in the coronary arteries.

Realistic geometry cartographic imaging

This is a Hungarian developed non-invasive technique. It takes 20 minutes (roughly) using a few disposable electrodes. Parameters are obtained using high precious data accusation system.

Pressure, volume, time of blood flow are collectively obtained by simultaneous recording, electro-cardiogram (ECG), phono cardiography (sound of the heart), non-invasive continuous blood pressure and trans-thoracic bio-impedance.

The acquired parameters are then mapped against a mathematical model and a cartogram is obtained, which is a collective behavioural pattern of the heart and its circulation status. This gives a complete hemodynamic picture of the heart, as well as the location and severity of coronary artery disease and relative oxygen demand of the heart. This imaging can detect coronary tube blockages as low as 20% and has more than 92% sensitivity and specificity (as claimed by the developers).

The main aim of this article on the non-invasive techniques for heart patients is to create an awareness about why a doctor asks you to do these tests and how exactly do the reports help in diagnosis and treatment of the disease.

The RGCI is still very new and needs further evaluation and cross checking before it becomes a tool for diagnosing and treating heart disease.

Angiography: excessive commercialisation

Angiography is an overused investigation being done more often to push the patient to the table of bypass surgery or angioplasty than to diagnose the extent of heart disease. This invasive and expensive test can find out the extent and the position of the blockages, but in a very inaccurate way. The test should be done only on those patients, who wish to undertake bypass surgery or angioplasty. Many non-invasive and safe tests already exist, which can diagnose the presence and extent of coronary heart disease (ECG, exercise stress test or TMT, thallium, spiral CT, RGCI etc). Even a patient's symptoms are good enough to diagnose the disease roughly.

One must remember that until the blockages are more than 70% in one or more arteries the heart disease will not surface at all. And once it sets in, diagnosed, confirmed with an ECG or TMT — it is very clear that the blockages exist (more than 70% at least). Now, if the patient chooses to follow only medicines or life-style changes or both it is not useful to get an angiogram. On the other hand, if the patient has decided to opt for bypass or angioplasty then the angiography test is indicated.

But due to commercialisation of cardiology in our country or abroad, most doctors/cardiologists insist on angiography to the patient, even when there is no doubt about their being heart patients. They persuade heart patients to undertake this expensive test, on the pretext of finding out the existence of the blockages, while they already know that they have crossed 70%. It is mostly used to put fear into the patient's mind and compel them to go for angioplasty or bypass surgery.

Most of the patients agree to take angiography because they are not told about the complications and consequences of the test. They are told that the test is very safe and it is only to confirm if the blockages are at all there. Many patients, when they agree for angiography, feel that the blockages may be 15-20% and this will clear them. But the cardiologists already know that there are more than 70% blockages.

But the real drama starts after the test is over. Even if the blockages are 70%, a cardiologist will say after coming from the OT (Cath lab to the people who know) that there are very severe blockages, and the only option left is bypass/angioplasty. The patient is in a dangerous condition and immediate action is needed. The patient can die any moment from a heart attack. Even if the patient takes it lightly, the doctors put the relatives in a panic, with a 'do or die' situation. If the blockages are even more than 80%-90% — whatever it may be — the same emergency is created. In the face of this fear and pressure most of the patients agree for an operation, spending their hard earned money of lacs of rupees.

I have come to hear and see that these cardiologists do not explain anything at length or allow any discussion about the validity of these operations, chances of re-blockage after operation, causes of the blockage, cholesterol etc. They put the fear and push off. The patient's relatives (wife, son, brother etc.) who thereafter cannot discuss anything with the doctor, have to agree, even if they have to borrow the money.

The patients, if they are told of these possibilities in the beginning, would never agree for angiography. Almost all would refuse. So most of the private hospitals follow step-by-step procedure to make the patients incur so much expenditure.

If the patient plans to postpone the decision, many hospitals refuse to discharge him. They put more pressure by emphasising that the patient's condition is very serious and it will be at their own risk. And the risk is of death!

I know many of my colleagues in the medical profession will not be happy with these facts, but most of the patients would agree as they have already gone through this ordeal.

Not that the cardiologists do not feel bad about this fear and commercialisation, but they have to run the infrastructure, where crores of rupees have been invested. No other operation can give so much money in medical science. The pressure from the hospital mounts. The doctor also knows, if he does not do this, others would still use these tactics.

Many cardiologists can deny these facts, but these are common things that are happening. In India nobody agrees that he is corrupt, but corruption is rampant. People are aware of it.

Angiography: the procedure

In angiography, a long wire called catheter is inserted inside the artery of the leg, near the thigh crease. This catheter is then pushed against the blood flow towards the heart blindly. With a view of the tip of the catheter on the fluoroscopy monitor (which exposes the patient to heavy radiation) this catheter is pushed onwards by trial and error method. If it gets stuck somewhere on the route, it is withdrawn a little and again pushed in. Not only does it scratch the whole length of the arterial tubes of the body but it can also puncture any corner of the tubes. Once the tip reaches the heart area, further manipulation is done to push the tip into one of the coronary arteries. Once inside the coronary tube, after a lot of trial and error, a radioactive dye is injected through the hole in the catheter and further fluoroscopy photographs are taken.

The tip of the catheter is withdrawn again, negotiated inside another coronary tube and the same photos are taken.

If the dye seems to fill up the coronary tubes completely, the blockages are probably not there. If the dye cannot fill the tubes (as roughly seen in the photos taken) inside, it is taken as filling defect and indirectly interpreted as blockages. The viewer mostly puts a rough percentage.

This report, being an eye estimation is given as 70%-80% and so on. It varies from one viewer to another. It also depends on the timing of the photograph (best is before the dye is washed out), angle of the photograph etc. and is thus amenable to a lot of different reports. It is not at all accurate and thus given in variations of 10%. One of my patients came to me the other day and told me that in the last two days he has already reversed his heart blockage by 10%. I asked, "By what method"? He said, "The second cardiologist, told me that the blockage was 70%. It was 80% according to the first cardiologist!"

Cured yesterday of my medicines, I died last night of my Physician.

— MATHEW PRIOR

Complications of Angiography

1. **Death**
2. **Myocardial Infarction**
   Factors predisposing
   Unstable angina
   Angina at rest
   Recent sub-endocardial MI
   Insulin dependent diabetes mellitus

3. **Neurological**
   Transient
   Persistent (stroke)
   A-V fistulae
   Haematomas with vascular and neural
   Compression
   Delayed haemorrhage

4. **Local, Brachial and Femoral Complications**
   a. **Brachial**
      Arterial thrombosis
      Median n. injury
      Late arterial bleed
      Bacterial arteritis
      Local cellulitis, phlebitis
   b. **Femoral**
      Arterial or venous thrombosis
      Distal embolization
      False aneurysm

5. **Perforation of the heart or great vessels**
6. **Vaso-vagal reactions**
7. **Arrhythmias and conduction disturbances**
8. **Phlebitis, infection, fever**
9. **Pyrogen reaction**
10. **Hypotension**
11. **Allergic Shock**
    Hypotension/anaphylaxis

12. **Other Complications**
    Pulmonary oedema
    Pulmonary artery perforation
    Pulmonary haemorrhage
    Coronary artery dissection
    Cholesterol embolization
    Systemic or pulmonary embolization of vegetations
    Pulmonary embolism
    Catheter entanglement
13. **Drawbacks**
    High costs and risks involved
    Invasive procedure

Accuracy of Angiography

All the time you must have noticed the blocks are reported on 70%, 80%, 90% and so on. Why should they jump by 10% each time! This only shows how rough estimates are generalised and made a round figure. Ten to twenty percent variations are also there depending on the individual bias or variability of the cardiologist concerned. Angiographies are casually performed in India in most hospitals and are highly inaccurate.

Diseases usually confused with heart disease

A. *Gastric pain, gastritis, oesophagitis:* Commonly known as gas problem or gastric pain, these can mimic the symptoms of angina. Many angina patients avoid going to the doctor and do not take any precautions as they are ignorant of the manifestations of angina. Association of breathlessness, radiation to arms, relief of pain with rest or Sorbitrate, sweating, choking sensation are the hallmark of angina whereas gastric pain usually manifests itself as burning sensation, spasmodic in nature and does not aggravate on exertion.

B. *Muscular pain in the chest muscles:* There are muscles on the chest which can be easily injured or sprained. If this occurs on the left side of the chest it may often confuse the patient. Such pains may be relieved by applying pain ointments like Moov, Iodex, Elgipan, etc., or by having pain killers. There is usually a history of muscular pull or injury.

C. *Cervical Spondylosis:* Cervical spondylosis is also a stress related disease and it manifests as shoulder pain, left or right arm pain and chest pain. The difference is that cervical pain is continuously present in both the right and left side simultaneously and is relieved by pain killers (and not with sublingual Sorbitrates). It is also recommended to confirm cervical disease by an X-ray.

The remedy is worse than the disease.

— Francis Bacon

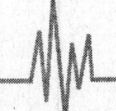

Heart Attack and How to Avoid It?

Contents

What is a heart attack?

Heart attack or myocardial infarction (medically called MI or coronary thrombosis) is the consequence of the complete ob-

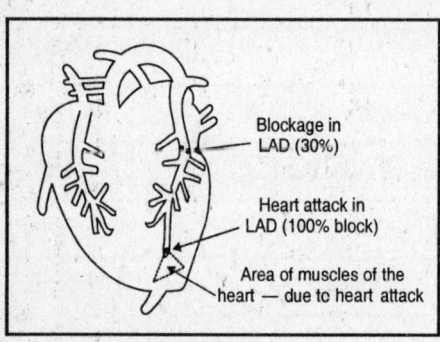

Blockage in
LAD (30%)

Heart attack in
LAD (100% block)

Area of muscles of the
heart — due to heart attack

struction of blood supply to a part of the heart muscles. This occurs due to a 100% blockage in any of the coronary arteries or their branches. The heart muscles are completely deprived of their blood and oxygen supply which leads to death.

The severity of the heart attack would depend on how much area of the heart muscle is actually involved. It is mild, if only 5 to 10 % area is involved and most of the patients survive. But if the dead area is more than 30 to 40 % of the heart muscles, the attack is considered severe, and if not managed properly and immediately, can even lead to death.

What is the cause of the heart attack?

Almost all heart attacks are sudden in onset and the cause is a rupture of the growing blockages. The blockages are usually covered by a thin membrane called intimal membrane, which also keeps the deposits intact. This elastic membrane gets stretched as fatty deposits increase. But if the fatty deposits continue below this permeable membrane, one day the time will come, when the membrane cannot stretch further and breaks off. This leads to the formation of a clot or thrombus inside the tube, closing the lumen completely. This completes the process of the heart attack. The area of the myocardium (heart muscles) which gets blood through the closed artery, dies in the event of no blood supply.

Heart attacks, often occur after a heavy meal, full of fat, sudden anger or excessive sorrow or grief or excessive stress. Heart attacks occur more frequently in the early mornings.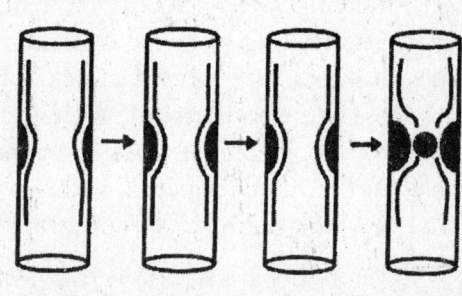
Heart attacks also occur during the process of angiography and angioplasty when the catheter or balloon is inflated and completely blocks the lumen of the coronary artery or breaks off the blockage by mechanical means.

Absurd — how has heart attack been accepted?

If the above is the cause of the heart attack, one can easily interpret that the sole cause of the heart attack was the growth of the fatty blockage in majority of cases. If the growth of the blockages is not allowed, the covering membrane would never burst. What should ideally be done by any doctor, is an advice to modify the risk factors of heart disease, by eating low fat food, regular exercise, stress management, yoga, weight reduction, control of high blood pressure and diabetes.

Unfortunately, this advice is not given by cardiologists and big heart institutes. Most of the doctors have accepted the fact that one day or the other the heart attack has to come. So rather than prescribing the proper life-style they prefer prescribing only symptomatic medication. More often they accept this eventuality. I don't know whether this helps them in their practice or not, but it will never help the patients who continue to suffer.

Surprisingly, the patients have also accepted the fact that even after taking all these medicines and undergoing surgery they may still have a heart attack. There is a general tendency amongst heart patients to ask their cardiologists for their residence or mobile phone numbers so that in case of a heart attack they can reach the doctors without delay. They do not know that they may not have a heart attack if they completely change their life-style.

There is no such thing as an accident. What we call by that name is the effect of some cause, which we do not see.

Prevent heart attack completely

The diagram and the above paragraphs, give the clue to the prevention of heart attacks. The simple message is: "Do not create more blockages. If you can reduce them, heart attacks would never occur."

It is like a bundle of notes tied with a rubber band. If you keep on putting more and more notes inside the rubber band, one day the rubber band has to snap. This is the situation of a heart attack where the membrane also snaps. If you stop putting more notes, the rubber band will never break. Further, if you start taking out one or two notes from the bundle everyday, the rubber band will never break.

The same principle applies to the prevention of heart attacks. Control of all the risk factors of heart disease by an adequate change in life-style can prevent heart attacks. The following are the expected parameters to prevent heart attacks :

1. Cholesterol 130 to 160 mg/dl

2. Triglycerides 60 to 120 mg/dl

3. HDL cholesterol 40 to 60 mg/dl

4. Blood glucose (fasting) 70 to 100 mg/dl

5. Blood glucose (PP) below 140 mg/dl

6. Blood pressure 120/80 mmHg

7. Maximum permissible exercises

8. Body weight in proportion to height

9. Stop smoking completely

10. Control stress

11. Oil/ghee in food is banned completely

12. Consume salads and fruits in plenty

13. Restrict consumption of milk/milk products

14. Avoid meat of any kind.

The object of preventive medicine is to enable people to die young as old as possible.
— ERNST L. WYNCER, MD

If you have a heart attack

I would not have added it to this particular chapter but ultimately decided to do so, because people who did not know about SAAOL earlier can also have a heart attack.

Symptoms of a Heart Attack

1. *Chest pain not relieved by rest or Sorbitrate:* The victim of a heart attack often complains of an excruciating pain in the left part of the chest, radiating to the left arm. The pain is

not relieved by taking rest or Sorbitrate (or other nitrates) below the tongue.

2. *Sweating:* This pain is often accompanied by profuse sweating. Even in a cold atmosphere the patient perspires.

3. *Feeling of intense weakness:* In many patients there is a feeling of intense emptyness or giddiness following a heart attack. Some of the patients often feel a low blood pressure and low blood sugar.

4. *Suffocation:* Choking, sense of constriction in the chest. There may be a feeling of breathlessness in some patients. Those who already have angina, would find an acute aggravation of the symptoms.

5. *Burning sensation in the chest:* This feeling occurs specially in people having a heart attack for the first time. This uncomfortable feeling, accompanied by a gastric or acidity problem, often confuse the heart attack victims. They consider this as a gas problem and take some antacid tablets, which also relieve the feeling to some extent.

Confirmation of the Heart Attack

Electrocardiogram: A simple ECG is the best way to confirm a heart attack. There are very clear cut changes in the ECG of heart patients having heart attacks. The ST segment becomes elevated, which confirms the attack. If there is a doubt about the ECG and the pain/symptoms continue, the patient should be asked to rest and the ECG can be repeated after an hour.

Blood enzyme tests: After the heart attack there is muscle damage, from where some enzymes are released into the blood. These enzymes, if raised, are suggestive of a heart attack. Some of these enzymes are called CPK, CPKMB, LDH, SGOT, SGPT etc.

Immediate Treatment of Heart Attack Patients

During the heart attack the muscles of the heart die, as they are not getting any blood supply. As the cholesterol blockages cannot be removed (which form 70-80 %), the blood clot removal is the only source of relief for the patients who are in the process of losing the heart muscles.

An immediate injection of clot busters like Streptokinase, Urokinase (very expensive injections) or drip of Heparin is the only possible remedial measure. If they are able to break the clot (which usually closes 20-30% of the lumen of the tube), the heart muscles would be able to get at least some blood immediately and will survive if administered within one hour of the attack. These injections can nullify almost all the damages of the heart attack. It still has some effect if given within five hours. But many a time these injections fail to deliver the results. These medicines also have their side-effects like internal bleeding, cerebral haemorrhage, peptic ulcer bleeding and can be dangerous sometimes.

The damaged area of the heart causes a strain on the other live areas of the heart muscles. And it is very essential to avoid further heart attacks. So, after a heart attack, the patients are advised to stay in the hospital for a period of about seven days, the first few days being in the ICCU (intensive coronary care unit). Here, it is possible to take care of any emergency.

Early mobilisation of the heart attack patient, starting from the fifth day, is the latest concept of treatment. Previously it was seen that heart patients were not allowed any movement for the next one month or so. Now the dictum has changed, as with early movement (walks, exercises) the recovery has been found to be quicker.

Assessment of the damage

What matters in a patient after a heart attack is the amount of muscles that have been rendered dead or damaged during the episode. The damaged or dead areas or muscles will not contribute to the pumping of blood from the heart, reducing the capacity of pumping. This pumping power of the heart (left ventricle which is the most important chamber) is called ejection fraction.

Echocardiogram is a test that can give an estimate of the pumping capacity of the left ventricle or the 4th chamber. It determines the ejection fraction (EF), which indirectly gives us the figure which has been damaged or dead. The normal ejection fraction is about 60%. If the EF after the MI or heart attack is 55%, it would mean that only 5% has been affected by the heart attack. On the other hand if this figure is 30%, this means it was a major heart attack and almost 30% of the muscles have been damaged. Please note that for bare survival even 15% ejection fraction is adequate. With 30% EF it will be possible to carry on with almost all the normal work.

Whatever be the damage, one must remember that the muscles which are not affected, need to be protected at any cost. The cholesterol deposits are there, even if the clot has been removed. One should work very vigorously to stop further accumulation of blockages and strive to reverse the existing blockages.

Aftercare of a heart attack

As a result of the heart attack, the initial damage done can be assessed after about 10 days and measurement of the damage gives an idea about the future needs. If the EF is more than 40%

or so, it is a safe thing. After three weeks the angina can be assessed with a stress test or TMT and after medication, life-style modifications can be made for future improvements.

If the pumping power is less than 40%, more care is recommended. The patient needs more medication and a vigorous life-style change on war footing. A regular visit to the cardiologist is recommended.

The need for angiography arises only when the patient is determined to undertake a bypass surgery or angioplasty. But these cannot revive the dead muscles.

The human body is the best healer. Though it cannot revive the dead heart muscles, the damaged tissues can be supplied with more blood and with adequate life-style changes, it is possible to revive the damaged muscles. This can ultimately increase the EF by 10-20%.

The past cannot be changed. The future is yet in your power.

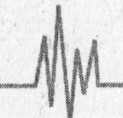

Section 6

The Present System of Heart Care

Contents

Health is not a condition of matter, but of mind. Nor can the material senses bear reliable testimony on the subject of Health.

— MARY BAKER EDDY, 'SCIENCE AND HEALTH'

How firm was my belief in medical science, and how medical drugs failed me

Let me explain what made me turn against the so called medical/cardiology science about 15 years ago. At that time I was a hard core medical doctor working in the department of cardiology in one of the prestigious hospitals of Delhi. I was just an MBBS, fresh and bubbling with the knowledge of medicines.

This confidence came to me because I had seen the wonders of the medical world. With knowledge of the human body, I could diagnose human ailments, confirm the clinical diagnosis with the help of ultramodern equipment and treat the diseases using drugs. I knew, if the diagnosis was correct, the treatment would also work, because the drugs have known roles and compositions. When, as a new doctor, I proved the efficiency of the power of using these tools to treat the patients during my internship and house job, I had no doubt about the usefulness and efficiency of the system. This gave me more confidence. When I worked in the children's ward during my internship in paediatrics in Kolkata, I diagnosed meningitis in a child who was about to die, confirmed the germs with a lumber puncture, gave Penicillin and Gentamycin injections, dramatically saving the child from an almost certain death. Without my help, the child may have died in no time. I saw the gratitude that the child's mother had in her eyes when the patient was being discharged. I knew what I was doing was 100% correct.

But everything broke down, in just one day about 15 years ago. All my confidence was brought to zero, like the fall of a castle made of playing cards. One of my patients helped me in knowing that all that I was doing to treat the heart patients, step. I wrote another three medicines, increasing the total number of tablets to nine. I sent him back with a fresh assurance that he will be okay this time.

After another month, he came back and was full of enthusiasm. He said he was leading a very normal life — working, visiting people, eating and had even played badminton one day without any problem. He was a completely normal person. He was so happy and even offered some gifts as gratitude. As a young doctor, I was moved by these praises and after some formalities of refusal accepted the gifts as a special case. When I wrote the prescription this time, I just wrote — repeat all the nine tablets. I was very happy with this gentleman. He was one of my favourite patients.

I showed these gifts to my fellow doctors with a lot of pride. I definitely was a good doctor. I was more confident now.

The next visit of the patient was not that encouraging, as he had the same pain again. I prescribed three more medicines. The total number of tablets per day was twelve after this prescription. I assured him that he will be okay. He was also very confident of my assurances. He knew that I would solve his problem again and expressed his satisfaction about my treatment abilities.

In the next visit, he had some more problems and I had to increase his dosage. When I sent him back this time, he was worried. I gave him my hostel room number and address so that he could contact me in an emergency. I prescribed in all fifteen tablets plus an advice to take Sorbitrate SOS (whenever required) below the tongue.

Nearly after ten days, this patient's wife woke me up early in the morning in my hostel. Her husband, my favourite patient was admitted in the emergency. He had an acute chest pain. I rushed to the emergency. He had a massive heart attack, Myocardial Infarction in medical language. I was very unhappy. Why was absolutely baseless and wrong. That changed my attitude and my life.

I was treating a patient in the Out Patient's Department. One gentleman came to me with complaints which were typical of a heart patient. He had a pain on the left side of the chest, while walking. This pain would subside if he slowed down or stopped walking. The pain would often radiate to the left arm. He also complained of breathlessness and a choking sensation, specially while climbing the stairs. I was almost certain about my diagnosis, he was a typical angina patient. I asked him if his symptoms were worse after meals, he said that on empty stomach he could walk 2-3 km but after a heavy meal the pain would come even after walking a hundred steps. My diagnosis was confirmed.

He was a heart patient, with blockages in the heart arteries. This I confirmed, as a standard procedure, with an ECG which showed the changes.

As usual I was very confident. I assured him that he was going to be alright and I prescribed him six tablets. There were three tablets of Sorbitrate, two tablets called Beta-Blocker and half a tablet of Disprin. I asked that gentleman to report after four weeks. I knew within my heart that this gentleman would have no problems when he comes next.

When he came next time, after about one month, he was full of praise. His symptoms had completely vanished. He could walk and climb stairs without any difficulty. He told me that I was a wonderful doctor and wondered how at such a young age I could treat him so well. I was 26 at that time. I was very happy and immediately prescribed the same six tablets to him and told him to continue the same treatment. He would have to report after a month again.

On his second visit he was having the symptoms again. The same pain and breathlessness. I took no time to decide the next had this happened to this patient who was doing so well? He was so happy and had offered me so many praises. Why did he have to suffer?

Somehow I managed to get him a bed in the ICCU (Intensive Coronary Care Unit). He was shifted immediately. We put him on continuous-ECG monitor. One after another injections were given to him to stabilise his heart. His heart suddenly started behaving badly, we gave him an electric shock. He recovered again. It was like a tug of war between life and death. I was deeply upset. Not that I was not used to this scenario, but this was my favourite patient. In the next three hours it was a crisis and ultimately the patient died in front of my eyes.

I was shocked. My best patient died. I was feeling guilty. May be my initial treatment was wrong. Why did he have a heart attack? Why did he die? I took all his papers to the duty room and started analysing. What was my fault? I matched all the medicines and found them in order. I had made no mistakes according to the medical textbooks. It was not my fault. I was again confident, after discovering that it was not my fault that the patient died. The books cannot be wrong. Medical science cannot be incorrect.

But the agony would not leave me. His eyes, his stares when he was dying were constantly haunting me. His praises and his trust in me. And still he had to die. I started thinking again that night. I started to put together all the events one after another. And suddenly I discovered a blunder. A perpetual blunder that I was committing!

I suddenly realised that it was I who had killed this patient. He had blockages in his arteries when he came to me for the first time. My diagnosis was correct. Coronary heart disease! His life-style and food was wrong, his blood pressure was high, he was always overweight and his cholesterol was also high. I did not bother except casually telling him to control them. I put more stress on the medicines. As his condition improved he did not bother to control his life-style. The blockages grew gradually. I did not bother and indirectly gave him relief by suggesting more medicines. All through my treatment his blockages were growing with the deposits of more and more fat in the arteries. I just kept on increasing the dosage. Ultimately he suffered a heart attack and died. It was like a planned death.

The realisation made my stomach heave. I realised that if I had changed his life-style adequately, this doomsday would not have come. He died because my training was biased towards the medicines, rather than life-style changes. I was more concerned about giving him relief rather than a permanent cure. This kind of treatment only had one result — heart attack. If the blockages are allowed to grow, the heart attack must come.

Suddenly I realised that the whole lot of doctors in cardiology are doing the same. All the heart attacks that I see everyday are results of a similar maintenance job being done by the cardiologists. Alongwith the drugs prescribed the blockages keep on increasing. Almost all these heart attacks can be prevented, if the process of this failing maintenance with the drugs can be changed. This was not a treatment!

The more I analysed, the more I realised, that the present system of treatment with medical drugs was faulty. It is a temporary job, which cannot cure this disease where blockages grow everyday. This is a temporary maintenance. Then, what is the treatment? Why am I not doing the treatment?

My confidence broke down on that particular day. I realised then that the cardiology I practised was a faulty science. Instead of treating the disease, I had almost become a planner of death in cardiology. I could also make out the difference between the treatment that we offer in case of infections. When we give antibiotics to kill the germs we actually treat the disease, thereby curing the patient. Once cured the patient does not require drugs. This is true in case of meningitis, pharyngitis, pneumonia, diarrhoea and so on. Medical science is wonderful then. As a doctor you actually treat, because you eliminate the cause of the disease. If the cause was germ infection, then what were the causes in heart disease? And that day I got the first clue that helped me to gradually develop a new system of treatment over the next 15 years.

In later years, I saw unnecessary bypass surgeries and angioplasties being performed by doctors. They refused to see reason. You have to work to cure the disease from the root and stop its growth. If the disease grows, the tubes which they replace or clean, are again going to get blocked. If you accept this fact, please go ahead with a temporary maintenance.

In the next few pages I am going to discuss, in detail, how the present system of treatment (actually maintenance) is only a short-term relief. A relief that has no consideration for the cure of the disease. The disease just goes on endlessly. The real treatment lies in a life-style change. At times I may repeat some of my observations but they are only to re-emphasise what I want to bring out.

Many doctors and cardiologists who read this chapter may feel offended as I have tried to point out the drawbacks of the present system. But they cannot deny the facts. Yet, if they are also adequately advising their patients on life-style, along with the maintenance job with drugs or surgical relief that they usually offer — they should not feel guilty or condemned. I also use medicines for my patients to offer them relief, but I withdraw the same medicines once the disease is at such a stage where the relief comes on its own.

Medical science –a powerful tool with basic faults

Medical science has done tremendous progress over the years.

It has now become a synonym for treatment. Combined with reasoning, proof and research, the application of this science has spread all over the world. Accepting modern technology, medical science has improved its efficacy, and the quickness and use of computers has made it even more advanced. The regular use by a large number of people, so called patients, helped medical science gradually to build a huge infrastructure. People then, in large numbers, wanted to become medical doctors. Soon medical colleges came up and with the number of medical doctors increasing with time, medical science has emerged more powerful and a completely accepted system of health care.

But there was a snag. Medical science tried to repair the human machine but faulted in its maintenance. Instead of informing people about what to eat, what not to eat, how to exercise or maintain a healthy body, medical doctors concentrated more on repairing the body only when things went wrong. Without proper knowledge as more and more people got ill, medical science tried to solve the problems by using medicines and surgery. This artificial creation of crisis and then a solution at the time of crisis made medical doctors more important. They enjoyed the importance and conveniently forgot the maintenance part. This went on. People suffered due to lack of knowledge and got diseases; the doctors and surgeons did good business.

They used more medicines and opened more operation theatres and hospitals. Medicines helped some infections and controlled them to a good extent. But most of the diseases like coronary heart disease, diabetes, arthritis, cancer, high blood pressure which were

> Medicine of the future will not look only for a one-to-one correspondence between an individual and a disease, will not separate body, mind, and spirit, will not only find broken parts and mend them, will not be an isolated approach. Medicine of the future will treat the person in the context of environment and social and cultural atmosphere. It will take the will and the belief system seriously.

not due to infections, continued to increase. Pharmaceutical companies took over the medical science. Then medical research mostly meant how to develop new drugs which earned more profits for them. The basic research and dissemination of information on maintenance of the human body took a back seat. This is the fault with medical science. They are knowingly allowing the human machine to get ill, while maintenance is gradually forgotten.

Suffering people gradually realised the discrepancy of medical science. When health care budgets of governments went up, they also did a retrospective analysis and found that the preventive aspect had to be given much more importance. The US Federal Government took a lead towards these aspects. The non-governmental organisations also projected the same faults in medical science.

Public awareness suddenly grew all over the world, almost exponentially. More and more people started looking at medical science and its proponents, with a little suspicion. They started searching for an alternative system which is oriented towards solving the problems permanently, without invasion or side effects of drugs.

Stay away from doctors and stay out of hospitals. An extraordinary proportion of the people in hospitals are quite ill, so obviously they are not suitable places for people who wish to be well.

— REUEL A. STALLONES, DEAN, TEXAS SCHOOL OF PUBLIC HEALTH

The fabulous human body machine — the best in the world

I consider myself a mechanic for the human machine. Just to learn about this machine I spent about five years in the medical college before I was declared qualified to treat it. This was my MBBS course.

During those five years we were taught in the first and second years the subjects of anatomy and physiology. This was only to make us understand the human machine and to know its functions. We used to open the dead and discarded human machines (dissection classes) and learn how beautifully they were built — we were taught how lacs of components like the brain, eyes, ears, liver, heart, stomach, bones, bone marrow, lungs, arteries, veins, nerves, muscles and tendons, pancreas, thyroid, spinal cord, joints (the list can just go on) constituted the body and how beautifully they were packed in such a small space. We learnt about how the machine was created from the fertilisation of the egg in the mother's womb to the birth programmed to expand over the first 18 years or so (till the child grows). It took more than 500 days of morning to evening classes to learn about the basic anatomy of the human body which was just about one tenth the size of a car. It is indeed the world's best machine, unparalleled, of course.

I could never realise this during the time I was doing my MBBS. I was just learning these as I wanted to become a doctor. All I knew was that if I study for five years I shall get a degree called MBBS and I will be able help a lot of diseased people and will be respected and so on. I knew that my parents will be happy if I work hard and stay in medical college and pass all the examinations at the end of the course.

After passing my MBBS, I spent 15 years of my research with the human body and only then realised the beauty of the machine. How magnificent the machine is! A machine designed to last for 100 years with billions of components!.

In physiology we were taught the functions of these components — how each one of them works in harmony with the other. Some of the similar looking components work together to form a unit. Lacs of these units form a larger component called the organ. Few of these organs form an organ system and then the body ....

> Knowledge is power.
> — THOMAS HOBBES

I realised that I was very interested to read about this particular subject — how the body functions normally. Why does the heart pump blood and supply the exact amount of blood to different parts of the body at rest and during exercise? How does the intestine absorb all the fats and cholesterol that we eat and store? How does the brain think and react to stresses? What effect do stresses have on different organs and so on. How does the body repair itself? This was probably the real foundation of the SAAOL in my mind.

In biochemistry (one of the subjects in the first one and a half years during MBBS) we were taught the chemical structure of the body. The composition of food that we consume. The chemical structures of cholesterol, triglycerides and how they are produced inside the body. The calories, carbohydrates, fats, proteins, their structures, requirements, functions, metabolism, all were taught to us one by one in this subject. I realised this knowledge was more vital for me in my later career, as I started to advise people to choose their food habits.

I believe that the first one and half years are the most vital part of a doctor's training. The soundness of this knowledge is what makes a good doctor. If we use this knowledge to keep the body healthy and also to repair it, it will be the best medicine.

The smallest structure of the body is a cell. It is so small that we cannot even see it without the use of a powerful microscope. There are about 100 billion (10,000 crore) or more such units in our body. These smallest units of the living body need food and oxygen in proper proportion to survive individually. They can obtain their survival energy from their own powerhouse called the *mitochondria*. The nucleus is their brain which decides every action. These tiny units can as well replicate themselves i.e. produce children, exactly similar to themselves (cell division).

A lot of progress is being made in medical technology, but

we have yet not been able to manufacture a single cell of the human body by using the advanced scientific technology, leave aside the organs of the living body.

I do not know who has actually built the human body, who has planned it so immaculately. If the knowledge of evolution is to be referred, then it has taken billions of years to produce the human being from a single crude cell. According to the theory of evolution the first living structure was a single cell like amoeba. It gradually advanced and duplicated itself to produce a multi-cellular organism. Millions of years passed as this happened. I am just referring to a table to let you realise how the single cell has progressed to evolve into a human body.

If you compare these figures of millions of years with the development of human science, which is only a few thousand years old, then one can realise that there are still miles to go for medical knowledge i.e. the science of the human body to reach perfection.

At this point, let me also add that what we do in the next three years of the medical career is to use this knowledge to diagnose and treat the disease using only medicines or surgery or both. At some places where it involves killing of bacteria/germs with chemicals, medical science has done a remarkable service. Where there is an accident or defective building of the body, surgery has proved to be highly effective.

YEARS OF DEVELOPMENT OF THE HUMAN MACHINE		
Earth was created	-	460 crore years
Single cell organism	-	150 crore years
Multi cellular organism	-	70 crore years
Fish-like animals	-	55 crore years
Reptiles	-	40 crore years
First mammals	-	25 crore years

Birds	-	20 crore years
Dinosaurs	-	15 crore years
Monkeys	-	10 crore years
Human types	-	1 crore years
Modern humans	-	1 lac years
Agriculture developed	-	10,000 years
Harappa and Mohenjodaro	-	3,500 years BC

But where there is a defective maintenance of the body — by eating wrong food, lack of exercise, man made excessive stresses or a smoking, use of medicines or surgery cannot compensate. The cure has to come from a change in the underlying defects.

Preventive cardiology

Preventive cardiology is one of the less practised branches of cardiology and is widely looked down upon by the cardiology community. There have been a few reasons behind this. The first was that the subject was taken very lightly and the approach was too mild to be effective. Reduction of the risk factors was not clearly defined, the approach was half-hearted and there was absence of adequate literature. Whatever books were available, they were meant for doctors and not for the people who had to practise these. Most of the available literature was epidemiology and discussions without clear instructions for patients. Preventive cardiology got a step-motherly treatment, as the cardiologists' orientation was more focused on medication, which did not cure the disease but gave immediate relief to the patients. After the advent of surgical interventions like bypass surgery and angioplasty — this important branch of preventive cardiology was more neglected, not only because the results were very slow, but also because it was in direct competition with the surgical approach.

Recently, there has been a slow revolution. The cost and complications of surgical treatment on one side, and the increasing awareness about preventing heart disease by the patient community, led to a fresh demand for a new brand of non-invasive cardiology — aggressive preventive cardiology. The aim was not only prevention but also cure. To be accepted by the patients, this method had to be highly scientific, practical and the results of the treatment had to come in a short period so as to convince the patients to follow the treatment further.

One must understand, when I talk of heart disease I refer to the coronary heart disease — the most common of the cardiac ailments today.

Increasing Number of Heart Patients

In the last few decades, in spite of a revolutionary technological progress in medical, interventional and surgical divisions of cardiology one thing is clearly apparent — the number of heart patients is increasing. Today, it is accepted that India has a dangerously increasing number of heart patients — the number can be anything between 20–50 million.

This signifies a gross failure on the part of the present practice of cardiology. Apparently, the growing number of big cardiac centres and heart institutes are not the scorecard of success but failure to control the disease. If the number of heart patients is increasing in spite of the so-called progress in cardiology what is the effectiveness of the present approach?

To search for the actual reason, one has to look at the real cause — the risk factors of the coronary heart disease. With the large-scale lack of knowledge about food habits, decreasing level of exercise, unrelenting promotion of cigarettes and so called healthy oils and the increasing stresses of modern life, the number of heart patients has grown to the present level. So, the answer remains in solving the causes and adopting a realistic approach. This approach is aggressive preventive cardiology.

Faults in Preventive Cardiology

Preventive cardiology, till now has described the risk factors of coronary heart disease with a range. The range included the highest to the lowest limits of a particular risk factor. Since it is convenient, most of the patients tried to maintain themselves on the highest level of the normal range. For example, the defined range of serum cholesterol is 130 mg/dl to 200 mg/dl. Most of the patients who have about 200 mg/dl feel very happy and consider themselves completely safe. As an aggressive preventive cardiologist, I would recommend them to bring their cholesterol to 130-140 mg/dl. The idea is to look for the best possibilities. If you can reach the bottomline of all the risk factors, prevention definitely is at its maximum and often leads to a reversal of the disease.

The second problem of preventive cardiology is the absence of improvement. This is what patients need in order to follow recommendations. Till now, the recommendations have been mild, the results had also been only preventive and not a cure — which the patients need and expect. Many of the cardiologists or doctors would consider slow progress (compared to a fast progress of the blockages which leads to an infraction or heart attack) of blockage as prevention. Even after following the previous instructions, people would still get heart attacks and no improvement, breaking their determination to follow the advice after sometime. Mild to moderate changes were not enough to make them complain in the long run.

The aggressive prevention aims at reversal and not just slow progress or no progress. Now it is a proven and accepted fact that the blockage can be reversed. Even if the blockage goes down by 1-2%, there is a tremendous symptomatic improvement and the patients are completely protected from a heart attack.

The third fault of preventive cardiology is lack of importance given to stress and its management. Though today stress is considered as the major reason of heart disease, because of its non-measurement (in terms of clearly defined units like kilograms, milligrams or millilitres etc.) the medical science has not given proper importance to this most important parameter. Stress management again has not been included in the control of heart disease. This needs to be done immediately.

The fourth and the main fault of preventive cardiology is the absence of practical instructions and guidelines for the patients. Most of the instructions are ambiguous. When we know that oils are triglycerides or fats are the apparent cause of arterial blockages, then these should be clearly forbidden. If our body requirement is 10% of the calories from fats and is obtainable from invisible fats present in cereals and other food that we consume, we should clearly instruct no intake of any oil (or triglycerides) for heart patients. This alone is not enough. We should also teach them how to cook food without oil and yet make it tasty. In the absence of a viable alternative the instructions become redundant.

Therefore, the need is not only clear instructions, but also evolution of a complete package, which can be followed by the community in a practical way. This should not be confined to one or two risk factors but should include all the possible risk factors of heart disease.

The time to repair the roof is when the sun is shining.

Medicines which do not cure

Here I am going to discuss the medical drugs which we use to give relief to patients. During this discussion I am going to describe the functions of the drugs, their mechanism of action and side effects. The information has been simplified, avoiding scientific jargon, to make the readers, who are mostly lay persons and heart patients, understand the broad perspective. They should not try to use these medicines on their own and should always refer to doctors who are qualified to advise them about medicines. The science of cardiac pharmacology is a huge subject, consisting of a lac (1 million) of pages and those who have done medical studies for ten or more years to study them can never be equalled. This is broadly to apprise them about the medicines for their knowledge.

Till date coronary heart diseases are being treated with drugs (medicines) which result only in a temporary relief from symptoms. These, under no circumstances, bring about a permanent cure as the cholesterol blockages in the coronary blood vessels are left unaffected. In other words they act only to maintain the disease condition. The effects last only till the drug is in effective concentration in the blood and gradually this concentration decreases and the dosage needs to be repeated.

As a matter of fact, this is a problem with the medical treatment as patients feel that they have improved and remain ignorant of the simple fact that these blockages continue to grow in size as the volume of cholesterol deposition is not controlled.

Most of the drugs used in the treatment of coronary artery diseases bring about temporary relief of symptoms through the following actions:

> Both physicians and the patients must come to terms with the inability of medicine to postpone death indefinitely.
> — Leslie J. Blackhall, MD

1. *Vasodilators*: Some medicines dilate the coronary

blood vessels, thus, increasing their luminal size and bringing about an increase of blood supply through them. These drugs have a duration of action, may be only a few hours and when their effectiveness is over the coronary blood vessels once again attain their normal size by shrinking. In order to maintain the dilation, another dose has to be taken.

2. *Blood thinning drugs:* These drugs reduce the viscosity of blood. In other words they thin the blood, thus more blood which is thinned is able to pass through the narrow space between the blockages. These drugs are widely used to prevent clot formation inside the heart tubes.

3. *Drugs which reduce the oxygen demand of the heart:* There is a further group of medicines which reduces the oxygen demand of the heart thus enabling the heart to do more work with the compromised quantity of blood which it is receiving due to blockage.

4. *Anti-cholesterol drugs:* These drugs prevent the release of triglycerides in the blood, lowering its level. The effect of these drugs is only till the drug is being taken and the fall in the blood triglyceride level is not permanent.

Nearly all the drugs used by cardiologists to treat coronary heart disease are selected from one of the above groups, and from our understanding of their mode of action it is appreciable that all of them bring about a temporary relief to the symptoms, while leaving the blockage as it is. In fact, they add considerably to our disease by their side-effects. In the meantime the disease gradually grows. Our medication is consequently increased with no cure. Soon the rosy picture fades away and once again we find ourselves back to where we started from, and we realize that drugs used in the treatment of CHD are primarily directed to the increment in the reduced blood supply of the ischaemic myocardium (muscles of the heart). All these drugs have their effects at certain levels of concentration in the blood. As these levels reduce along with their excretion, the drugs are no longer capable of producing their beneficial effects and the doses have to be repeated once again. At the moment there is no drug that has any action on the cholesterol blocks, hence, benefits of all the drugs in the treatment of CHD are temporary.

If the whole materia medica, as now used, could be sunk to the bottom of the sea, it would be all the better for mankind — and all the worse for the fishes.

— VOLTAIRE

DILATERS/NITRATES

Drug names	Side-effects
Angispan Sorbitrate Angitab/Monit Monotrate Imdur Ismo Vasotrate Nitrofix Angised Isordil Nitrocontin	throbbing headache, nausea, flushing, weakness, sweating, palpitations, dizziness, fainting, blood disorders.
Nikoran, Zynicor, Korandil, Corflo	
Trivedon Flavedon, Cytogard, Metagard	

BLOOD THINNING DRUGS

Drug names	Side-effects
ASA 50 Asprin Ecosprin Ticlop Dynasprin Cardiwell	Gastro-intestinal discomfort, nausea, vomitting, hot-flushes, skin rashes, vertigo, cholestatic jaundice, dizziness, diarrhoea, headache, hypotension, tachycardia
Elopidogrel, Ceruvin, Deplatt, Clopivas, Plagril etc.	

Nevertheless, the implication and judicious use of drugs is mandatory in the treatment of CHD and these should never be discontinued without prior advice from medical practitioners.

Drugs which reduce the Oxygen demand of the heart

The drugs which come under this group are further subdivided into (a) calcium channel blockers (b) beta-blockers (c) ACE inhibitors. Drugs coming within this category reduce the oxygen demand of the heart muscles, thus, enabling the heart to do more work with the compromised amount of blood it is receiving due to the blockages.

a) *Calcium Channel Blockers:* Calcium is essential for the contraction and working of the heart muscles. The more the calcium entering the heart muscles through channels in the muscles, specially the slow calcium channels, the more it beats at a higher rate. This in turn increases the demand for blood and oxygen by the heart muscles, the supply of which is already compromised by blockages in the coronary arteries. The drugs in this group, as their name suggests, block the entry of calcium through the slow channels into the cardiac muscles, thus, slowing down the heart rate and reducing the demand for blood and oxygen by the muscles of the heart.

b) *Beta-blockers:* These drugs also block the action of receptors on the surface of the heart muscles which when stimulated cause an increase in the rate of beating of the heart and in turn, an increase in the demand of blood and oxygen by the muscles of the heart. When these receptors are blocked, the rate of beating of the heart is reduced, thus, enabling the cardiac muscles to manage with reduced supply of blood.

c) *Angiotensin converting enzyme inhibitors (ACE inhibitors):* Angiotensin is a very potent constrictor of blood vessels. When a blockage is already present, the lumen of the coronary arteries is substantially reduced, and if there is further constriction of the coronary arteries, with blockages present in them it will

CALCIUM CHANNEL BLOCKERS

Drug Names	Side-effects
Nifedipine	Dizziness,
Calcigard	headache,
Depin	weakness,
Myogard	nausea,
Nicardia	peripheral-
Veramil	oedema,
Isoptin	palpitation
Dilcontin	and nasal-
Dilzem	stuffiness,
Nifelat	ischeamic pain,
Angizem	rashes,
Kaizem	tachycardia
Dilcardia	
Amlopress	
Stamlo	

BETA BLOCKERS

Drug Names	Side-effects
Atenolol	Hypotension,
Betaloc	bradycardia, cold-
Tenormin	extremities,
Betacard	headaches,
Aten	dizziness,
Antecard	nightmares,
Lopresor	angina, fatigue,
Betabloc	constipation,
Betacap	indigestion,
Metolar	wheezing, ankle
	oedema, nausea,
	flushing,
	impotence, skin
	and eye reactions,
	jaundice, gingival
	hyperplasia,
	gynaecomastia

ACE INHIBITORS

Drug Names	Side-effects
Newace	Hypotension,
Enapril	angio-
Envas	oedema,
Aceten	renal failure,
Listril	headache,
Lipril, Cipril	hyperkalemia,
Cardace	fatigue,
Remace	dizziness, GI-
Losar	Upset, cough,
Losacar	decreased
Angizàr	white blood
Enace	cells

result in a complete occlusion of the coronary arteries and ob-struction of the blood supply through them. Here below is a brief mention of a few drug names (trade names) from each of the above groups responsible for reducing the demand of blood and oxygen by the heart.

Half of the modern drugs could well be thrown out of the window, except that birds might eat them.

— Martin H. Fischer

Anti-cholesterol (hypolipidaemic) drugs

ANTICHOLESTEROL
(Hypolipidaemic drugs)

Drug names	Side-effects
Simvotin	GI-Upset,
Simcard	impotence, skin
Lipistat	rashes, headache,
Aztatin	painful
Rovacor	extremeties,
Zocor	blurred vision,
Lopid	cholestatic
Bezalip	jaundice, angio-
Normlip	oedema,
Pro HDL	pancreatitis, atrial
Tripid	fibrillation, non-
Lovostatin	cardiac chest pain,
Lipizyl	diarrhoea and
Lipigem	vomitting
Lipistat	
Lovastat	
Storvas	
Atocor lipicor	
Atorlip	
Tg-tor	

Drugs in this group reduce the levels of VLDL (very low density lipoproteins) and triglycerides in the blood. They prevent the secretion of VLDL from the liver.

Drugs from each of the above groups which are em-ployed for the treatment of coronary heart disease are initially necessary but they are never free of side-effects, which occur due to prolonged use. Here below is a list of the most com-monly used drugs from each of the groups mentioned along with their side-effects for your understanding.

All substances are poisons; there is none, which is not a poison. The right dose differentiates a poison and a remedy.

— Paracelsus

The surgical interventions for coronary heart disease

Over the past few decades surgery has held a key position in the management of coronary heart disease.

The surgical management of coronary heart disease involves two widely performed procedures — percutaneous transluminal coronary angioplasty (PTCA) and coronary artery bypass grafting (CABG). These procedures have been popular and give dramatic and immediate relief from angina. This euphoria gradually diminishes as time passes. It has been further explained in more detail.

Surgical treatment of coronary heart disease can be of the following types, though these are temporary in nature and are unnatural methods to solve the symptoms.

A. Coronary artery bypass surgery (CABG)

B. Coronary angioplasty (percutaneous transluminal coronary angioplasty, PTCA)

C. Coronary angioplasty with stent implantation

D. Other angioplasties:

 – Directional atherectomy

 – Rota-blading

 – Laser angioplasty

E. Other surgeries:

 – Minimally invasive CABG

 – Heart transplantation

The greatest single curse in medicine is the curse of unnecessary operations, and there would be fewer of them, if the doctor gets the same salary whether he operates or not.

— RICHARD CABOT, MD

Some common stories of my patients

To begin with, let us see a small sample of heart patients who came to us to join the SAAOL Heart Program in the first few years of its inception. (All these are true examples, but due to professional ethics I have changed the names of people and places).

Case No.1

Prof. Shankernarayan, 64, had been a very important person. Apart from heading an institution for 15 years he had many outside assignments, had written many articles. He was a man on the move. Though he had controlled his weight, maintained a reasonable level of walking (despite being a very busy person), just after his retirement he started having a peculiar constricting pain in the chest. Initially he ignored it, but he had to stop walking whenever the pain occurred. If he carried his overloaded briefcase (which was full of papers, pens, stapler etc.) the pain would come within 20-30 metres of walk. After meals it became impossible for him to walk. He told this to his wife. Both of them went to see their personal physician, Dr. Gupta. Angina pain was confirmed by the physician and that he had developed blockages in the coronary arteries. He was put on medication.

Professor Shankernarayan and his wife decided that they could not wait any further. He could not afford a health problem because he was getting busy again. So many meetings to preside over, he had to travel all over the country to take interviews for important posts. One day he was in Delhi, next day in Mumbai and the following week in Chennai. He was on an important committee of the Government and had to visit China. He decided to solve the problem immediately.

> I am dying with the help of too many physicians.
> — ALEXANDER THE GREAT

His personal physician organised an angiogram. He was informed of the risks of an angiogram but there was no option. His wife signed the consent. The film showed one major blockage in the left anterior descending artery (LAD). The cardiologist wanted an immediate angioplasty or ballooning and said without that the risk would be very high. There was a panic but the wife was not convinced. One week went by.

Looking at his busy schedule and important assignments, the professor agreed to undergo an angioplasty, which the cardiologist said would remove his heart disease. He will be a normal man again. A hefty fee was not a problem for him. The ballooning was done soon and he was discharged from the hospital after two days.

He started walking again. The pain disappeared. The family breathed a sigh of relief. His normal routine was resumed.

Within a month the pain reappeared. The constriction in the chest was similar. They visited the same cardiologist. They were told that the blockage had redeveloped in all probability. Another angiogram was needed. Medicines were restarted. The fear came back. Professor's wife was more concerned. Their children staying in the United States were very worried. They could understand the temporary nature of the treatment, being scientifically oriented. They wanted to know the reason for the blockage, and why did the blockage redevelop?

Professor Shankernarayan was about to go for another angiography when he came across an article on the SAAOL Heart Program — about changing life-style. He was not impressed but somehow he decided to meet the doctor.

In October, 1995 Professor Shankernarayan cancelled his appointment for the angiogram and joined a three day resort program organised outside Delhi.

Case No.2

Mr. G.P. Saxena was always on the move, being a busy executive. In 1989 he had angina, and a bypass surgery was immediately done as the angiography showed blockages, which the surgeons thought were very dangerous. Mr. Saxena had no other option but to go in for surgery. The only consolation was that the doctors assured him that it will be a permanent solution and for at least the next 15 years he will be free from any problem. Three grafts were carried out in his heart.

Mr. Saxena went back to work soon after the surgery, with a big chest scar and a long cut in both the legs, from where the veins were removed for the grafts. In 1993 he felt breathlessness again. The angina was confirmed by a stress test which was positive. The surgeon suggested another angiography. Reluctantly Mr. Saxena had to agree. This time he was told that two of the tubes were blocked again and a new block, which was 50% in 1989 was now 80%. Another bypass surgery was the only solution. After a few more opinions he agreed to undertake the second bypass surgery. This time the grafts were taken from the chest arteries and also from his hands.

Mr. Saxena was further given about six kinds of medicines which he was supposed to have everyday. Without any question he had to accept the tablets though the surgery was successful.

Mr. Saxena was told that he was over-weight and the cholesterol was a little up, but nothing to worry about. He decided to undertake daily walks as a precaution but continued to eat fish, chicken etc. which the doctors had kindly allowed. They took TMT tests every year thereafter. By 1998 his TMT was positive again and his cardiologist advised another angiography to check again. Mr. Saxena realised that once again he had the same problem.

Case No.3

Roshan Lal Agarwal, a businessman based in Mumbai, used to smoke a lot for years. He also had a lot of stress being in the transport business. When he developed some burning sensation in his chest and breathlessness, he did not think he could be affected by heart disease. Instead of changing his habits he went to a naturopathy hospital for sometime and he felt better. When he came back again his sons insisted that he visit a cardiologist, as was suggested by the family physician. Mr. Agarwal was very confident that he did not have a heart disease. But after being pressurised by the family he yielded to their demand and landed up in a prestigious hospital in Mumbai.

The cardiologist told the unsuspecting Mr. Agarwal that he would need a small test called angiography to confirm the heart disease. Mr. Agarwal knew something about the invasive nature of the test and since he was living with problems and leading an active life he was not agreeable. But the persistence of the cardiologist and his sons (who met the doctor separately) somehow again brought him to the hospital to get the test done. He just wanted to know if something was wrong. A long catheter was introduced in his leg artery and after a few hours he was moved to the hospital room. He was relaxed and was really keen to know the result.

In the evening the cardiologist announced that Mr. Agarwal had a blockage of 80% in one of the very important arteries and he wondered how he had been saved from a heart attack till now. The cardiologist said that if he did not get a small operation called angioplasty done, his life would be in danger.

I had my money and my health. I strained my health to get more wealth. I spent my health to get more wealth. I lost my health and my wealth.

Seeing no way out and observing the fear in the eyes of the family members, Mr. Agarwal agreed for an angioplasty with stent (a small spring like device costing Rs. 50,000 each) without delay. Though he was completely against any invasive procedure he had to submit himself. Somehow the ballooning was done and he was discharged after a day with a discharge slip that he has been treated for his blockage. Now the danger had been averted and he could go back to work. The family members were very happy and thanked the doctor who did the angioplasty. The cost was Rs. 3,75,000, which was within the reach of the Agarwal family. Mr. Agarwal, who was totally against the surgical treatment, was still not completely satisfied but was at least happy that he would be able to go back to his business.

Within two months the burning sensation and breathlessness returned. He and his family did not expect such a possibility. He was rushed to the same hospital. The cardiologist, after hearing all the symptoms feared that there may be something wrong with the stent. He asked the patient to get admitted for an angiography. Mr. Agarwal could not think of it and he was not ready for the second angiography. By this time he had talked about his heart disease to many people and knew a little more about the disease. He insisted with the cardiologist for a stress test, where without angiography one can know about the reblockage. He came back home.

The burning sensation persisted. The sons again convinced him to get admitted to the hospital for the test where the second angiography was performed. Mr. Agarwal was told that there were two more blockages — one each before and after the blockage, apart from the original blockage.

The doctor said that he could not be discharged from the hospital since his life was again in danger. The risk of heart attack had returned.

The worst had happened to him again. The doctor suggested that he could still control the risk if he submitted for a new technology of

> The remedy is worse than the disease
> — Francis Bacon

angioplasty. It could be solved only by a bypass surgery or a new procedure where the doctor will open the blockage with a Rota-blade and fix two more stents, one before and the other after the old stent. Since Mr. Agarwal was completely against a by-pass surgery, after a lengthy discussion the family agreed for the new technique.

The next day the new procedure was done. The cardiologist congratulated the family waiting outside the cathlab. Though it was a very difficult procedure, the doctor was successful. There was a sign of relief. The cost for the operation this time was Rs. 6,00,000. The next day he was discharged. He was supposedly back to normal again!

But Mr. Agarwal was never normal again. The complaints never disappeared completely. He had the burning sensation again. The fear was back. The person who could challenge his sons, at the age of 60, to work as hard as he did, was not the same. The courage had gone. He was a broken man always think-ing about his heart and the blockages. Two angioplasties and Rs.10 lacs brought him down with the same problem again.

In 1999 he joined the SAAOL heart program to reverse heart disease.

Any interference with nature is damnable. Not only nature but also the people will suffer.

— ANAHARIO

Angioplasty: plumber's Temporary solution

Percutaneous transluminal coronary angioplasty (PTCA): When one or at the most two coronary arteries have significant block-ages which are constantly impeding the blood flow to the heart and the patient has symptoms of angina, such as chest pain which may radiate to the arms, tightness in the chest, choking in the neck or breathlessness to name a few, then this procedure is generally preferred.

In this procedure a catheter is introduced under local anesthesia either through a blood vessel in front of the elbow (brachial approach) or through a blood vessel at the loin (femoral approach). This is then guided into the heart under radio graphic observation and placed at the mouth of the coronary arteries. From within this catheter another balloon tipped guide wire is introduced and the balloon is positioned at the site of the atheromatous (cholesterol containing) blockage. The position of the balloon is confirmed by a contrast angiography. Then the balloon is inflated with a radio-opaque material which facilitates its visualization. The balloon is inflated a few times in order to press the blockage to the sides of the coronary artery and achieve a wider lumen through which more blood can pass, under angiographic observations. Then the catheter is withdrawn. It is now a common practice to insert a spring or a stent at the site of the ballooning to check the blockages from collapsing into the lumen of the coronary artery. The patient is then kept under observation to see whether the dilated segment remains stable.

Hospital admission is necessary for this procedure and the patient has to undergo various investigations and is also put on medication to facilitate the procedure.

Complicated and expensive, PTCA is a highly invasive procedure and is not without serious drawbacks. It is not a permanent remedy as the blockages are not removed and the deposition of cholesterol continues in the coronary arteries and is left unarrested. Reblockages are very common and occur within 3 to 6 months. New methods of angioplasties such as stenting, laser angioplasty, directional atherectomy or rota-blading do not have the tremendous advantages that they are supposed to have. The basic process of reblockages is again related to a wrong life-style and damaged intima of the blood vessels. For the sake of reference and knowledge, some of the complications of PTCA are mentioned below:

1. Injury to the coronary arteries.
2. Bleeding at the site of the ballooning.
3. Coronary artery tear.
4. Formation of out-pouchings (aneurysms) in the weakened walls of the coronary arteries.
5. Sudden closure of the artery leading to a heart attack.
6. New clot formation (thrombus) in the coronary arteries.
7. Heart attack.
8. Irregular heartbeats (ventricular fibrillation).
9. Sudden cardiac arrest.
10. Complications from the dye that is used for angiography still remain and is dealt with elsewhere.

Comment is free but facts are sacred.

— CHARLES P. SCOTT

Bypass surgery: a road destined to close

Coronary artery bypass grafting (CABG): Coronary artery bypass surgery is another expensive surgical procedure which is a more extensive, mutilating and aggressive process of temporary solution to coronary artery disease. In this operation, the chest is opened in the centre in front. Blood vessels from the leg are surgically removed and used to bypass the coronary arteries which have cholesterol deposits (blockages) in them. In males, as there are no breasts, an artery of the chest is available (internal mammary artery) which may also be used in the operation. The operation is extremely complicated and intricate, and can also have serious and fatal outcome. The heart's function is maintained by a sophisticated machine known as a Heart Lung Machine. The procedure leaves a mark by a huge scar running down the front of the chest, and one on the leg. Although, with the help of this procedure we are able to bypass the blockages in the main coronary arteries and their major branches, by no means can we operate on the smaller branches of the coronary arteries which also contribute extensively to the reduced supply of blood and oxygen to the muscles of the heart.

Definitely bypass surgery is an abnormal procedure and cannot be an exact replacement of the original. The reblockages would again occur within a gap of 2 to 12 years with an average of 5 years. Those who do not follow a proper life-style can even get a reblockage within a year but those following a very good life-style would not get a reblockage for even 15 years.

Complications of CABG

1. Respiratory complications

    Alveolar dysfunction

    Pulmonary oedema

    Infection

    Phrenic nerve injury

    Prolonged ventilatory insufficiency

2. Post-operative hypertension

3. Heart attack (myocardial infarction) during operation

4. Cardiogenic shock

5. Left ventricular failure

6. Cardiac tamponade

7. Septic shock

8. Arrhythmias

Atrial fibrillation

Atrial flutter

Ventricular fibrillation

9. Blood clotting disorders

10. Wound infection, non-healing of wound

11. Peripheral vascular complications

12. Renal failure

13. Gastro-intestinal complications

Bleeding in the stomach, duodenum, shock liver syndrome

14. Reblockages

15. Damage the brain during the heart-lung machine running the blood supply to the brain.

Comment : After surgery (CABG) when someone gets a reblockage after 5 years and gets angina again — it is clear that the blockage is already more than 70% or more. Now suppose this 70% had developed in 5 years — i.e. 14% per year of reblockage. Many people accept it as a normal thing. This may also be calculated as more than 1% reblockage in a month after bypass surgery. How absurdly people still accept ongoing blockage — even after bypass surgery and still do not consider a life-style change!

Some interesting experiences of patients

1. Cleaning the tubes every years

One interesting patient joined our program after getting three angioplasties. He said, "Sir, these days every year I get the tubes cleaned from inside."

2. Emergency postponed for a month

It has become a common system to suddenly create an emergency after the angiography is done. Patients and their relatives are suddenly told they must get operated in a day or two. Unnecessary fears are put to pressurise the decision. One patient commented, "Sir, this was also the same with me. They told me and my family, that I immediately needed bypass surgery — it was almost an emergency. When I expressed my inability to organise the money for the operation before one month — they immediately postponed the emergency. I was told to come after one month with the money."

3. Why PTCA or ballooning is so costly!

One patient asked "Doctor, during angiography the catheter is already inside the coronary tubes — why can't they just introduce it further and inflate the balloon? Why do another catheter introduction — and why so much money for just inflating the balloon? The doctor replied, "Angiography is for Rs.10,000/- and for ballooning is Rs.1,10,000/-. Just the balloon inflation cost is Rs. 1 lac?"

4. How many angiographies are possible?

One inquisitive patient asked me, "Doctor how many angiographies can be done on one person?" I did not know.

But I met one special patient who had undergone 17 catheterisations under angiography procedure over the last 10 years. Can you imagine!

5. Medicated stent

Angioplasty has changed over the years making it more and more expensive. Everytime the old procedure fails — a new one is introduced. Initially it was plain angioplasty. It failed. So the 'stent' or spring was introduced in nineties. This also was found to fail as people blocked the stents in no time. Then came medicated stents. Within the next few years this also had to be changed. I am already seeing the failed results. The costs of these stents are exorbitant — but suits the cardiologists/hospitals. A stent costs Rs.50,000-70,000. Fabulous! And you coat it with a drug — the cost goes to Rs.1.5 lacs. One coating costs about Rs.1 lac! God save the heart patients.

Irony is that all the three are used now (though they have failed) as the money is good. All doctors and manufacturers of balloons and stents are happy!

I got the bills for my surgery. Now I know what those doctors were wearing masks for.

— JAMES H. BOREN

The SAAOL Concept

Contents

The meaning of SAAOL

SAAOL — stands for Science And Art Of Living. It is the best combination of modern medical science with the ancient arts. The name justifies the meaning.

SAAOL has another wonderful meaning. It is a very common Rajasthani word, which means 'to do things in the best possible way' or 'perfection'. Whatever you do should be the best or perfect i.e. SAAOL.

The name SAAOL was suggested by one of my cousins, Sanjay Jain, who stayed in NewYork city in 1994. Both of us know Marwari (a language widely spoken in Rajasthan) and the word is so common. It occurred so naturally. We just discussed and derived the 'Science And Art Of Living' meaning.

Today I am sure that SAAOL is really the best or perfect. It is the best (SAAOL) combination of modern medicine and the ancient art of yoga, meditation, stress management education about heart disease and dietary management. The more I think of the meaning of SAAOL the more it appeals to me.

The theory of SAAOL

SAAOL believes that the body is a unique machine which can run for a hundred years if we provide it with a proper environment. Though it can adapt to little changes in its maintenance, fuel, stress and strain, on prolonged misuse the machine gets damaged. But this machine is also unique in the sense that it can repair its own damages. This is unlike most of the man-made machines like cars and computers, which cannot repair themselves. Once damaged, man-made machines either need replacements or repairs from outside. The body is much superior to these machines.

SAAOL utilises this unique feature of the body. It provides the body with the best environment to help in the repair process. The blockages of the heart arteries have developed because we were eating wrong food, excessive fats, not exercising our body and giving the mind more burden than it can handle. SAAOL attempts to undo these factors by a combination of providing correct knowledge and training the human body to correct these mishappenings.

SAAOL does not consider the body as a simple combination of different organs which can be separately treated — as is done by medical science. It believes that the whole human body is a single unit, each of the organs is interactive and interdependent. We cannot take an individual organ approach to treat such a body. SAAOL subscribes to the theory that if you disturb one organ it will also have an impact on the others. Emotional disturbances of mind will also affect the stomach and damage the heart; the chemicals (medicine for example) given to help one organ would damage the other. It wants to dissociate itself from unnecessary medications. SAAOL takes a holistic view of the body.

The art of healing comes from nature, not from the physician. Therefore, the physician must start from the nature, with an open mind.

— PARACELSUS

What does SAAOL do?

SAAOL provides information and training to keep the body healthy and to remove diseases, especially the heart disease. A team of experts in cardiology, medicine, nutrition, yoga, meditation and process of stress control work under the same roof with a similar frame of mind. Patients and people who want to prevent heart disease are admitted for a few days along with their spouses in a small group to learn the theory and practice of the Science And Art Of Living.

The training deals with a detailed theoretical explanation about wrong life-style practices and their remedies; physiology of the human body and the pathology of the diseases and how in our practical life is it possible to implement this theoretical understanding. It also provides a complete practical training on health rejuvenating exercises and yogic practices to help the heart in its repair. The SAAOL Heart Program training gives equal importance to stress control in our practical life. The training gives a complete model for stopping the production of stress, release of stress and lastly management of stress. Nutrition and diet form another important component of SAAOL's training for heart patients. Besides providing all practical ways to calculate the calories of food, balancing different types of nutrients, SAAOL also provides practical training to cook tasty food without the use of any kind of fat.

When two do the same thing, it is never quite the same thing.

— PUBLILIUS SYRUS

Inception of SAAOL

The word SAAOL was probably chosen while I was in New York discussing about starting this new system of treatment with my cousin Sanjay Jain in December, 1994. He too is a philosopher. We wanted to give name to this program which was most appropriate. At that time I was working with the All India Institute of Medical Sciences (AIIMS).

> Progress is impossible without change and those who cannot change their minds cannot change anything.

We both agreed that since it has both the ingredients of science and art, we should have a name which will actually mean both. Hailing originally from Rajasthan in India, both of us know the Marwari language very well. Further discussion led to the name SAAOL.

The inception of the idea, of using something like SAAOL, for a medical doctor like me, who knew nothing except modern medical science, goes back to about twelve years. I had passed my MBBS and was working in the department of cardiology in a Delhi hospital. Death of a dear patient whom I was treating (now I realise it was maintenance and not treatment) for angina led to a sea change in my attitude as a doctor. He came to me for treatment of angina and I prescribed some medicines. After taking the medicines he improved immediately. Both the patient and I felt good about the improvement because the complaint had vanished. Within a few months I had to increase his medicines a few times because the pain reappeared. Every time I increased the number of tablets he reported a tremendous relief. Then one day he suffered a massive heart attack and passed away in front of my eyes.

While analysing the cause of his death, which gave a severe blow to my conviction as a doctor, after a spell of successful treatment with medicines, I looked for the reason responsible for that. As a believer in the theory that "everything that happens must have a reason."

I started analysing. I asked myself: Why did he die, if I was giving the correct treatment? When the answer came, I was shattered. The patient was actually increasing his blockages during the short spell of 'successful treatment' with drugs, which I gave him. He was eating meat and chicken, ghee and butter, leading a high stress life-style. He was also overweight. Thus

> When you encounter difficulties and contradictions, do not try to break them, but bend them with gentleness and time.

the deposits of cholesterol and fat carried on and I kept on prescribing more tablets to maintain the relief. Suddenly I realised that I was not treating the disease but was busy in maintenance of relief from angina pain. He died because I could not tell him that if he did not change his food habits and stress, the blockages would grow and grow. I could have done that. I almost felt that I was responsible for his death. I could have given him advice to change his life-style but I did not.

That blow was severe enough to make me question against the wisdom of the powerful and established medical science and the proponents of the science of cardiology. I found myself against everybody in the field because, I explained that what is being done by most of the cardiologists is not a treatment but a maintenance. This maintenance was sure to lead to a heart attack — it's only a matter of time as the blockages were growing. It is in fact a failure maintenance.

I asked too many questions. I was not practical, because I was questioning the popular system of writing prescriptions for heart patients. How can one, who has graduated almost recently, challenge the ongoing system of the mighty science of medicine and surgery!

I started analysing again. I understood that the departments of medical science, which take care of infections with antibiotics, are probably doing treatment. They were killing the bacteria and leading to a cure. This can be called a treatment. If the disease is over after administration of medical drugs, it can be called a treatment. Most of the diseases like diarrhoea, bronchitis, pneumonia, malaria get a treatment because the disease is wiped away after successful administration of medications. It is a treatment.

But what about heart disease? The medicines have to be taken throughout one's life and still the disease would continue to grow. It cannot be called a treatment, it is a maintenance.

I realised that both maintenance and treatment should go on simultaneously. Thus the SAAOL concept was born.

In the next twelve years the concept grew. More and more ideas were added while I actually started developing a complete systematic program. Two years at the King George's Medical College, Lucknow (while I was doing my MD) and the next six years in AIIMS, New Delhi saw a lot of things being added. The fat-free food cooking concepts developed. What I had in my mind in September-October, 1995 gave shape to the present SAAOL Heart Program.

I started the Program independently after I formed the SAAOL Heart Centre in 1995, having resigned from the All India Institute of Medical Sciences.

Discovery consists of looking at the same thing as everyone else and thinking something different.

SAAOL over the years

The last 3 years have been very adventurous and successful for SAAOL as it was a completely new concept and more so because it worked diagonally opposite to whatever the common practice has been in the last few decades. Initially it was very difficult to convince people that it would work and I had to explain for hours to the prospective participants. Doing it in government hospitals was easy than it was in a private set-up.

But as time passed by things gradually became easier. Our fame spread by word of mouth and our ex-participants were so convinced and improved that they started recommending us to their near and dear ones. The media also supported us.

> To be persuasive, we must be believable, to be believable, we must be credible, to be credible, we must be truthful.
> — EDWARD R. MURROW

Lots of people who got reblockages after angioplasty and bypass surgery joined us, because they were left with no other alternative, and the SAAOL system helped them to improve.

Word spread and people from distant places came to join the SAAOL Heart Program. There were people from many states (Punjab, Haryana, UP, MP, Himachal Pradesh, Rajasthan, Bihar, West Bengal, Maharashtra and many more). Some also came from USA, U.K., Middle East, Nepal, Sri Lanka and even from South Africa and Kenya.

As the Delhi Program started doing well, we were requested by a lot of people to hold the SAAOL Heart Program trainings in different parts of the country. One of my patients, Mr. Bijur, from Mumbai was very keen and promised to help in organising everything for us in Mumbai. He surveyed all the nearby resorts for us in Mumbai which ultimately resulted in the first SAAOL camp outside Delhi.

MUMBAI: The first program started on 28th Feb., 1997. The response was very encouraging. I really felt that Mumbai, which has the maximum number of heart surgeries and angioplasties was full of people who were very keen to join us. Mr. Bijur, Mr. Babbar, Mr. Damani, Mr. N. Gir — all our patients in the Delhi camp helped us a lot. Mr. Babbar lent us his posh office on New Marine lines, Mr. Damani gave us his guesthouse and Mr. Bijur received all the calls from the prospective patients. The SAAOL family (we consider all our participants as part of the family helped us to organise the Mumbai camps. We had to hold another program after three weeks seeing the tremendous response. Now we have hundreds of patients. The programs are held in Lonavala/ Khandala area in the Biji's Hotels.

> The best test of truth is the power of the thought to get itself accepted in the competition of the market.
> — OLIVER WENDELL HOLMES, JR.

CHENNAI: After a splendid success in Mumbai SAAOL

soon spread its wings to Chennai. The first program was held there on 25th April, 1997. This program was special because this was the first non-residential program of SAAOL. Again the response was encouraging. The program was inaugurated by the Honourable Mayor of Chennai, Shri M. K. Stalin (son of the then Chief Minister of Tamil Nadu Shri Karunanidhi). The program was held in a Five Star Hotel, Park Sheraton. Gradually more programs were organised in Chennai. I found that many of our participants had come there from neighbouring states and cities to join us. Our programs had people from Karnataka, Tamil Nadu, Andhra Pradesh and Kerala. The subsequent visits showed that those who joined the earlier camps had also improved. Soon after we decided that the SAAOL Heart Program would have to be continued in the south. We now hold regular programs in Chennai, Bangalore and Hyderabad.

KOLKATA: When the SAAOL Heart Program went off smoothly in Mumbai and Chennai, we planned it in Kolkata also. We kept the Kolkata programs also as non-residential. The first program was inaugurated on 18th July, 1997 by the well-known Member of Parliament, Shri Somnath Chatterjee, at the Great Eastern Hotel in the heart of Kolkata. After the first successful camp, another was held with greater zeal. And now we hold regular camps in Kolkata at short intervals. I have a special attraction for Kolkata as this is the city in which I grew up.

CHANDIGARH: The beautiful capital of Punjab and Haryana was our next target. Since many people from this city had already attended our Delhi camps we had no problem there. One of our participants, Mr. Kulwant Singh and his family were kind enough to extend their help in organising the camp. The first camp was held in Hotel Mount View (a non-residential one) from 1st to 3rd August, 1997. The response was very encouraging.

BANGALORE : After a series of programs in Mumbai, Kolkata and Chennai, success brought us to Bangalore, the most expanding metropolis. I went for a lecture to Bangalore in Sept. 1997, and even with the sitting capacity of four hundred, people had to stand outside the hall and listen to my lecture. Then and there we decided to hold our camp and one of our patients, Mr. S.S. Prasad volunteered to help us in Bangalore. The first camp at Bangalore was a running success. We were completely full.

HYDERABAD : The city of the nawabs was the other metro to come under the shelter of SAAOL. The first program was successfully launched on 25th of June, 1998. The camp was held at Hotel Ramada Manohar, one of the most beautiful hotels of Hyderabad. The attendance in the camp was beyond our expectation. The credit for such a move goes to our patient, Mr. Adi Narayana Rao, who helped us in all possible aspects.

While we were in different metropolitan cities we observed a contrast in the risk factor profile of people who consulted us with heart diseases. Thus, we carried out a survey and found that the risk factors were different in different parts of the country. In Delhi it was non-vegetarian food, central obesity and stress. Mumbai had more heart patients whose main problem was stressful living. In Chennai the stress problem was not as bad, but the people there consumed a lot of coconut oil and oil products. We found that in Calcutta more heart patients smoked heavily and they had a sedentary life-style. Being a metropolitan city the distribution of risk factors was not quite marked in Bangalore.

A new scientific truth does not triumph by convincing its opponents, but rather because its opponents die. And a new generation grows up that is familiar with it.
— MAX PLANCK

Reversal of CHD — most rational and scientific treatment

The Concept of Reversal — How Scientific is it?

The most rational solution to coronary heart disease lies in a permanent process which not only arrests the progress of blockages but also reverses the same. Blockage occurs gradually over the years as cholesterol from the blood flowing through the coronary arteries gets deposited (due to the risk factors) in the arterial walls. These deposits are mostly soft masses of fat with connective tissues and are in a reversible phase. Cholesterol and fat being easily dissolved in the blood can be picked up from the blockages if we can create an ideal situation.

Creation of this ideal situation is what is required in order to slowly reverse the blockages. The SAAOL Heart Program helps and trains people to create that ideal situation. Cutting down of all the risk factors at a time with the carefully selected set of yogasanas, meditation, a perfect practically possible stress management program, complete education and understanding of coronary heart disease, cessation of tobacco intake and smoking and a food awareness — cooking training — directs one to a perfect life-style which can reverse the blockages. All these have to be done under the guidance of cardiologists, doctors, dieticians, yoga masters in order to avoid complications — which the heart patients are easily prone to.

All heart patients know a little bit about prevention and they try doing these without much accuracy and consistency, making them unsuccessful and submitting to the surgical treatment ultimately. Had it

> Because the newer methods of treatment are good, it does not follow that the old ones were bad: for if our honourable and worshipful ancestors had not recovered from their ailments, you and I would not be here today.
> — Confucius

not been happening, none of these patients would have gone to a hospital for an emergency case.

The SAAOL Heart Program has developed this expertise over the last decade after a lot of experimentation and efforts. Each and every patient joining the program in the initial stage has helped the program to gradually improve. Heart attacks and other complications have been extremely low.

The SAAOL Heart Program is not magic. It takes at least two weeks to show the first signs of improvement. The improvement also depends on efforts put in by the patient, his/her age, the stage of blockage, co-operation of the family members and so on. We now have some angiographies of our patients done after attending the SAAOL Heart Program which prove that blockages can be reversed.

Reading books is a good way of learning but cannot substitute for a practical training. Books with hundreds of pages — some of them very important but most of them are not relevant to the patients and difficult to understand. It is much more difficult to put into practice, whatever is written. Had it not been happening, every patient would have become a doctor by buying medical books — and learning whatever the doctors know.

Nevertheless, what helps definitely is the fact that when you have someone who can give you the information you need — not in a way that you do not comprehend and definitely not less than that you do not learn at all.

The only hope I can see for the future depends on a wiser and braver use of reason, not a panic flight from it.

— F. L. Lucas (The Search For Good Sense)

Dr. Dean Ornish and the complete proof

Nobody even thought that this particular second-year medical student of the Baylor College of Medicine, Houston, would one day be one of the greatest pioneers in the most effective and logical treatments developed for the cure and reversal of heart disease, America's No. 1 killer, which is growing to a considerable potential even in India.

Born and bred in Dallas, he received his preliminary education from a public school. His father was a dentist and was quite content by the thought that some day his son would follow in his father's footsteps. As it is said of the temperament of an achiever, he joined the Rice University at Houston and discovered that he was no longer the brightest student. He was so depressed that he even contemplated suicide, but as fate would have it an episode of glandular fever gave him the chance to reconsider, thus making him a pioneer in the reversal of coronary heart disease.

Like many others of his generation in 1972, he too sought the enlightenment of the Orient and under the wings of his *Guru*, the honourable Swami Sachidanand, he succeeded in connecting with his inner self and realized that the less he needed success, the less strained he felt. This led him to the connection between depression and heart. In 1977 he started researching on the causes of heart disease and the factors that could possibly bring about their reversal, while he was still a 2nd year medical student. For a very long time no one could see the potential in his work, and dismissed him as a young, inexperienced and foolishly idealistic. While he was still in his third year of medical school he received his first big breakthrough, with his introduction to Henry Groppe, an oil business consultant, who had a firm interest in preventive medicine. Dr. Dean Ornish formulated a plan of life-style changes which had four major disciplines, all aiming at an integrated attack on heart disease and its reversal as follows:

1. Stress management which comprised yoga, meditation, of

imagery and breathing exercises, all together for the duration of not more than an hour a day.

2. Light aerobic exercises and half an hour's walk.

3. He asked his patients to stop smoking.

4. And to adhere to a strictly vegetarian diet extremely low in fat content.

As it is truly said, that the greatest truths are the most simple, Dr. Dean Ornish's approach to combating heart disease and its reversal produced remarkable results. In 1989 he started publishing data showing that his 'Firehouse gang' as he preferred to call them, who were at one time very seriously ill, were in fact improving. This brought the attention of the world to his work and soon invitations to medical conferences began pouring in. He also received grants from many organisations including the U. S. National Institute of Health (NIH). The acknowledgement of the tremendous potential of this humble man's work will one day lead us to the development of a far better and advanced medical therapeutic approach to the cure and reversal of heart disease from which everyone can benefit.

Dr. Ornish published his first report as early as 1979. In 1983 in a report published in JAMA (Journal of American Medical Association) he proved the lowering of all risk factors of heart disease by following the life-style advised by him. He showed that the pumping power of the heart also increased in his patients. In 1990 Dr. Ornish received wide recognition after he showed angiographically a reversal of arterial blockages by his program. This scientific report was carried by the most prestigious medical journal — the Lancet. He was then frequently quoted in *Newsweek*, *USA News*, *Reader's Digest*, *Span* etc., some of the most recognised magazines. He showed all the proof of reversal when he used the latest medical gadget 'PET Scan' to prove his reversal theory. This scientific report was again published in the year 1995 by JAMA. The theory became much more popular and today Dr. Ornish offers his reversal programs in eight major hospitals in USA including Harvard Medical School, Boston and Beth Israel Hospital, New York City.

Dr. Dean Ornish's results are now widely accepted and the latest textbooks of cardiology have brought out a separate chapter on Reversal of Heart Disease. The latest edition (1997) of the most reputed text book of cardiology, one of the most popular and voluminous books in the medical sciences — The Braunwald's textbook writes elaborately about how Dr. Dean Ornish proved that blockages can be reversed.

You can only cure retail but you can prevent wholesale.

— BROCK CHISHOLM

How medical science Accepts a new discovery?

Whenever a new discovery is reported to the scientific world, they say first, "It is probably not true."

Thereafter, when the truth of the new proposition has been demonstrated beyond question, they say, "Yes, it may be true, but it is not important."

Finally, when sufficient time has elapsed to fully evidence its importance, they say, "Yes, surely it is important, but it is no longer new."

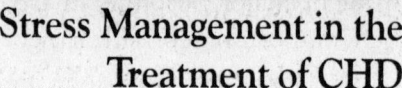

Section 8

Stress Management in the Treatment of CHD

Contents

contd....

Since you cannot build a life completely free from stress or even distress, it is important that you develop some ways of dealing with stress.

— NATIONAL INSTITUTE OF MEDICAL HEALTH

An angry man opens his mouth but shuts up his eyes.

—A CHINESE PROVERB

The importance of stress in the development of heart disease?

Stress reduction is probably the most important component of the SAAOL Heart Program for reversing heart disease. The word stress would mean tension, worry, fear, anxiety, anger, sorrow, lack of satisfaction and so on. A stressed individual may have one or more of these problems. But stress is probably the most important cause of heart disease.

If we analyse the causes of heart disease and look for the most important ones, we will find at least half of them are directly or indirectly due to stress. High blood pressure, diabetes, high cholesterol and smoking are directly related to stress and food habits (most stressed and busy people eat badly), lack of exercise (stressed and busy people don't have time to do exercise), obesity (due to lack of exercise and bad food habits they gain weight). Naturally, as we are talking of control of all these risk factors, stress becomes the most important one.

The irony is that till recently medical science has been neglecting stress management as a tool to treat heart disease. This was probably one of the most important factors that has led to the failure of the science of cardiology to control heart disease. In the presence of excessive stress, wrong eating habits, lack of exercise, smoking, high blood pressure, excess blood sugar, excess cholesterol deposit and smoking continued unabated. Everything went in the wrong direction.

To discuss why modern medical science failed to control the stresses of life — I have to offer some simple explanations.

In the last fifty years or so the problems of a fast life with technological advancements, increasing population, increasing demands, stiff competition, more work, less time and excessive inputs to the brain — all have increased the stresses of modern people. The overload of stress was the first reason for the lack of control over stress.

The second reason is due to the deficiency of medical science. It failed to understand the intricacies of the brain ('mind' in colloquial language) and its mechanism of action. Till today, the brain is the least known organ of the human body. The medical science now has been able to understand less than 10% of the brain structure and mechanism even with the spectacular technological advancement. More so it could not even measure or quantify the amount of stress. In the face of these failures, what could it do to control the menace of stress.

These are the two major causes which contribute to the failure of medical science to check common stress related diseases like coronary heart disease.

On the other hand, the Indian science of yoga and scriptures already had the technology to cut down the stresses.

Only recently, medical science has realised its deficiency as regards to stress and started its research of the oldest science of *yoga* and ancient Indian philosophy. Whatever little they tried to offer to control stress proved very primitive compared to the existing knowledge, as early as 5000 years ago. The behavioural science — the latest and the newest branch of modern medicine now speaks the same language of stress management. The psycho-neuro immunology (PNI) — latest development of medical science, now offers the same treatment of positive thinking and meditation.

Today it is apparent that stress management has become the cornerstone for treatment of heart disease.

Have a heart that never hardens. A temper that never tires. A touch that never hurts.

— CHARLES DICKENS

What is stress?

Stress is a universal word which is being used by just about anyone, wherever you go. A clear cut definition has not yet been evolved. Try to define it yourself and see what you face!

Medical science describes stress as a specific response of the body to all non-specific demands, be it physical or psychological, be it threatened or actual — the response being the secretion of ACTH and cortisol (these are two stress induced hormones). Secretion of two other hormones stimulated by stress are adrenaline and non-adrenaline.

A more practical definition of stress may be "when the problems presented by everyday life exceed your resources for coping with them, you feel stressed." But we must remember that stress cannot be imposed solely by external demands or problems but can also be generated from within, that is internally by our hopes, fears, expectations and beliefs.

Why most people cannot practice stress management

Stress has a multi factorial origin. It can come from anywhere — from work, family, society and so on; as well as from our interpretation of the realities of life. Our own understanding of the requirements for happiness and achievements can also cause stress. The way we communicate is also important in stress management. Ultimately, once the stress is created there are many things that can be done to quickly release it. There would still be stresses left, but they can be managed optimally.

Stress management is also like coronary heart disease, which needs complete intervention from every angle. Most of the managers of stress do not talk of this part. They talk about God and advise you on love but that's not complete stress management. Some would ask you to practise meditation or *Shavasana* —that again is incomplete. Advice on work-related stress management and so on are important but still not complete.

SAAOL talks about a complete model of reducing stress. It works on every situation. It offers solutions for everyone: for a layman, for a housewife, for a businessman, executive or retired person. For all of them stress management offered will work. If understood correctly, it can bring about tremendous change in life.

This complete model of stress management has one beautiful aspect; it can even make you successful in life workwise, moneywise and so on. Progress in these aspects of life is a must. You are not supposed to leave your work and then manage stress. This program is most suitable for busy people — those who have more work than they can handle.

Get good counsel before you begin and when you have decided, act promptly.

Why has stress gone up in the last fifty years?

1. Work Overload
2. Time Overload
3. Information Overload
4. Requirement Overload
5. Illness Overload

Work Overload means that everyone has to work more and more these days. Shopping, cleaning, telephone bills, children's study, their school, different taxes to file, bank accounts, TV repairs, car servicing, preparing food,

> From the errors of others a wise man corrects his own.

socialising, health check-ups, electricity, plumbing, making or receiving telephone calls, learning computer, reading, writing.... so much work has to be done that leads to an increase in stress. Fifty years ago most of these factors did not exist. People generally worked six to eight hours a day.

Time Overload means a chronic shortage of time, that is part of everybody's life in this modern busy world. The volume of work has increased. Naturally time stress has peaked up. Most of the stresses are because of the fear of getting late or lagging behind.

Information Overload. People are now overburdened with information. Even a child of four years is not spared and he has to read four to ten books. Adults have 40 pages of the newspapers to read, numerous TV channels and hundreds of books to go through just to keep themselves in tune with the modern world. The overloaded brain gets stressed.

Requirement Overload is another problem. Suddenly our re quirements have gone up. We want a fridge, TV, flat, cars, ten watches, twenty dresses, bank balance, air conditioners, designer sun glasses, ten pairs of shoes — the list is never-ending. To achieve them we need to earn more, work more and learn more. A vicious circle sets in.

Illness Overload is the last but not the least of the overloads. Due to a wrong life-style, no exercise and excessive stress every other person seems to have a disease, which leads to further stress. All these five factors can add up together and multiply each other.

Small stress reduction tip : Schedule daily uninterruptable organising time.

Sectors of life causing stress

Another factor for increased stress is the imbalance of the sectors of life. These are the particular areas, which when neglected, become responsible for all our stresses. Those who fail to take notice of these sectors and their importance, get stressed tremendously. These sectors are:

1. Money sector
2. Work sector
3. Family sector
4. Love and support sector
5. Ego sector
6. Social sector
7. Health sector
8. Spiritual sector

Money has become the most important cause of all stresses, as it is essential at every step of our life — survival, residence, food, needs, comforts, hobbies and then luxuries. Most of us mismanage the money sector badly. Some people have more money and some have less — but both have stresses of inadequacy. One must remember that inadequacy is not because of the amount involved, but because of the balance between the income and expenditure. If the expenditure or requirement exceeds the income of a person, stress is inevitable. To keep the money sector comfortable, it is advised to keep a positive balance between the income and expenditure. People must be self-sufficient and should not be dependent on anyone for their needs and expenditure.

After money is the *work* sector. For many, work or occupation is the main reason for stress. It may not be related to the hours of work, as I have seen many people working 16 to 18 hours a day and enjoying every bit of it. Work

> Small stress reduction tip : Make a list of tasks, in order of priority.

related stress only comes when one is not satisfied with what he does. If one does not like his work the stress becomes high. Work sector stress can be minimised if someone starts loving what he does — may be because of the salary he receives, satisfaction he gets, fame he obtains and so on. Each of them can cut down the work stress.

The *family* sector is also very important for one's stress. One of my patients complained that throughout his whole day's work he is enjoying, but the stress starts when he enters his home! The family plays a very important role in of stress for such people. Family should be the place to relax and not to increase stress. This is not happening in most families. One must remember that family is a social group and people should take keen interest in each other's activities in the family and help each other. It needs a lot of understanding, and good communication skills to have a peaceful and enjoyable family life.

Today family life is generating stress because we are becoming self centred and not taking interest in the likes and dislikes of the other members of the family.

Love and support sector also plays a very important part in stress production or its relief. Apparently, many people have wonderful families — with a beautiful wife, children, and grandchildren, all smiling in public life but there is often a lack of love among them. Rather than helping each other, sacrificing for each other, they are ready to harm each other. The love is gradually reducing. But there is a tremendous power of love in stress management. If

SECTORS OF LIFE

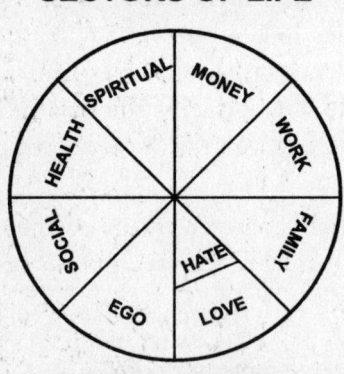

ARE YOU BALANCED?

one knows that family members will stand by him in the time of adversity, his love sector will be strong. This is gradually decreasing. The children are not dependable; doubts are there about unquestioned support from them. There is also an element of doubt about the wife, a fear that she may also leave in case of a crisis, is putting a tremendous insecurity on one's life. This can be vice versa also. This has already gone very bad in the western countries. Isolation, loneliness and insecurity are the main causes of stress in people's lives now. In India also it is worsening.

To improve the love sector, there is only one advice that I give to people. Help everybody without expectation of any return in exchange. Just help others to please yourself. It is the expectation that ultimately leads to erosion of love. You help someone, support him — not expecting back favours, the love sector would grow. Try it yourself and feel the difference.

Ego is the next sector. Many people have sufficient money, wonderful work environment, and well-knit family — ready to sacrifice for each other. The stress comes when one wants to show off at every moment of one's life — to boost one's ego. Trying to prove oneself in front of others, is an outcome of the ego. Excess of it is very bad. Ego cannot be contained if one knows one's shortcomings, faults, and smallness in the universe. Self-analysis and understanding of the realities can help in the reduction of ego. Ego is the hallmark of people who are insufficient, incomplete and ignorant. Exposure to spirituality can help them a lot.

Society, a group of people living in association, is also a stress booster. It is like a bigger family with fewer commitments to each other. Absence of a social life increases the deficiencies or the shortcomings of family life or love sector. A good social life, in other words, can make up for the other sectors. Having a

> Small stress reduction tip: Set realistic dead-lines.

friend, an associate, a social contact fills up the gaps and life becomes enjoyable. I suggest you make friends, visit clubs and recreation places, attend social functions, offer small help to others to have a good social life. This may help a lot. Isolation becomes more apparent in the absence of social life.

The *health* sector is also becoming a major cause of stress in modern society. Everyone seems to have one health problem or the other. Diseases have become a part of life. Excessive stress is now causing so many diseases that are known as psychosomatic diseases. Stress, thus caused by illness, can only be eliminated by a healthy lifestyle. Education about health should now become a part of the school and college syllabus. Knowledge about the correct food habits, regular physical activity and exercise, stress management training, yoga and meditation are the secrets of good health. Chemicals and surgeries are not the real answers for ill health.

The last sector about stress is the *Spiritual* sector. It can also be called the *moral* sector, for those who have little faith in God. A belief in spirituality, exposure to God's domain, can wipe out most of the stresses of life. I have come across many people who have failed in most of the sectors of life, but the spiritual sector has saved them. Submission to God, the Almighty, can cut down the stresses of ego, money, family, love and society. When I see a tremendous increase in the number of people going to spiritual organisations and temples and feeling happy and content, the answer is obtained. Belief in God can become a tremendous help in stress management. If you do not talk about God, remember morality. If you are morally sound, if you know that you have not harmed anyone, deceived your friends or family, there is a wonderful sense of well-being and satisfaction within you.

It is a good thing to learn caution from the misfortune of others.

Measurement of stress

How to Identify a Stressed Person?

I have met plenty of individuals over the years who do not agree that they are stressed. They simply cannot accept the fact that they have problems because they have not been aware of them. The success with money and an inflated ego sometimes does not allow them to concede.

The following are some distinguishing features of excessive stress:

Physical Symptoms

1. Tense muscles (shoulder ache, backache)
2. Irregular breathing
3. Dry mouth
4. Sweaty palms
5. Cold fingers
6. Knots in the stomach
7. Shaky hands
8. Frequency of urination

Behavioural Symptoms

1. Smoking
2. Tobacco consumption (e.g. *gutka*)
3. Repeated stimulant intake (e.g. tea, coffee)
4. Increased alcohol consumption
5. Nail biting, knee jingling, hair pulling
6. Reckless driving

> A person has two legs and one sense of humour and if you're faced with a choice it's better to lose a leg.
> — CHARLES LINDNER

7. Social withdrawal
8. Vacant look

Emotional Symptoms
1. Irritability
2. Short temper
3. Undue haste
4. State of anxiety
5. Feeling of depression
6. Irrational fear
7. Feeling of insecurity
8. Undue aggression
9. Sleeplessness
10. Bad dreams

Cognitive Symptoms
1. Loss of sense of humour
2. Loss of memory
3. Forgetfulness
4. Loss of common sense
5. Lack of clear thinking
6. Indecisiveness
7. Undue fear
8. Negative thoughts.

Well, one or more of the above may be the problem of people you associate with. Beware, they tend to bother you more on the days you are most stressed and disappear on days you are relaxed and not stressed.

Mentioned overleaf are some of the changes and responses

produced by the human body to stress. You will observe that maximum of these responses of the human body to stresses are harmful to the individual, his personal, as well as social and professional life.

Small stress reduction tip: Avoid indecisiveness.

Type-A and Type-B persons

Medical science and psychologists have now identified two types of people — one are very stress prone and the others who do not get stressed easily. They are known as 'Type-A' and 'Type-B' persons respectively. One can easily distinguish one from the other.

Type-A person is one who can create problems where there are none. He can create trouble where there is peace. The following are the identifying points of these two types. A person can be a varying combination of 'A' and 'B'. Yoga and meditation can change Type-A to Type-B.

Type - A

1. Always short of time
2. Rapid movements
3. Impatience
4. Polyphasic thought performance (proneness)
5. Tension
6. Restlessness
7. Preoccupied
8. Hostile
9. Forceful use of hands and fingers

> It is more important to know what sort of patient has a disease, than what sort of disease a patient has.
> — Sir William Osler, MD

10. Excessively critical of self and others

11. Tendency to use vulgar language

12. Rage, fury

17. Belief in inherent injustice

14. Competitiveness

15. Touchiness

16. Reactive

13. Dominating

18. Perfectionist

19. Punctual

20. Egocentric

21. Tendency for short time deals

22. Unable to delegate for fear of losing control

Type - B

1. Absence of Type-A habits

2. Absence of urgency and impatience

3. No free floating hostility

4. Lack of need to display or discuss achievements, unless the situation demands

5. Plays for fun and relaxation, does not play for display of superiority

6. Able to relax without guilt

7. Able to work without agitation

8. Co-operative with others

9. Gives benefit of doubt

10. Flexible

11. Respectful of other's integrity

12. Not afraid to admit mistakes

13. Gives credit to others when due

14. Encourages trust and openness in team efforts

15. Delegates authority as much as possible

16. Takes a break when fatigued

17. Not devastated by criticism

18. Tell-me-more attitude

Without your exercising any conscious control over it, your autonomic nervous system and all your body functions react vigorously to both stress and depression.
— C. NORMAN SHEALY, MD

How much stress is actually required?

Talking of stress management, I must warn you that you cannot expect to go to zero stress. That is an impossible target for any of us. Some stress is required for you to stay in this society and to fulfil your responsibilities. Without it you will become an outcast in society or have to leave everyone and stay alone.

Stress can be graded into four levels, for the sake of understanding, though any watertight division is impossible to make. As no measurement of stress is available, we cannot quantify stress. But the following grading can still be done.

1. Minimum stress

2. Optimum stress

3. High stress or sub maximal stress

4. Very high stress

Minimum Stress

This is representative of very low or almost zero stress. Staying in this society — where there are requirements, responsibilities and problems, this grade is almost impossible to achieve. On the other hand those who reach this grade, though they themselves feel absolutely happy, are considered as incompetent, lazy, irresponsible, unsuccessful and frustrated, by common people. Their output is almost zero. I do not want you to reach this grade, unless you do not care for anyone or may want to be a saint.

To my mind these kind of saints are also not seen these days. The sadhus and spiritual gurus, who run big organisations, are also in tremendous stress. If they also wish to go that way, they have to leave every hope of name and fame and go underground to do *sadhana* (complete submission to God).

Optimum Stress

This is the ideal stress level that I would recommend you to achieve. Stress should be there but not tremendous. You should be comfortable with the whole situation, as well as produce good work, meet your responsibilities, be reasonably successful in life, content with what you have, have a good relationship with everyone around you. This is the stage I want a heart patient to achieve, in order to produce a reversal of disease.

To my mind about 10-15% people in modern society are keeping themselves at this grade. They are really happy. They probably do not need most of the techniques written in this book.

Small stress reduction tip: Consider each problem in depth.

High Stress or Sub-Maximal Stress

Most of the people in today's modern and busy society are in this state. They either aim too high vis à vis their capacity or are mis-managed or both. This is the point where stress related diseases start. They are good but their happiness level is low. They suffer from fatigue and exhaustion at the end of the day. They are still not satisfied and content. Still they feel as if they are trailing behind.

Almost 50-60% of people in the modern world, specially in cities, are in this grade of stress and need stress management. They also suffer from heart disease, as they keep on increasing the blockage. They must bring about more changes in their food, exercise more and educate themselves in order to stay disease free.

Very High Stress

This grade is the worst of all, but unfortunately many of us are in this grade. Too much stress, too much work, too many problems from every angle are the hallmark of this stage. They are hardly able to manage this much pressure and are often frustrated. They start making mistakes, behave badly (in spite of their non-willingness). Their output goes down. Heart disease and other diseases take over. This group needs SAAOL stress management on an urgent basis.

Description of human performance curve

Work or performance and stress are related. The above description can be interpreted in the following curve and the work
output of a person can be found out. See for yourself.

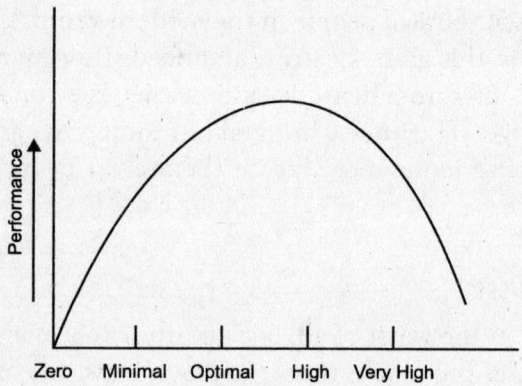

*Optimal or little stress is very much the need
of society and is recommended for a healthy
and productive life.*

Effects of excessive stress
on the human body

The Following are the Effects of Stress on the Human Body

1. Heart rate increases
2. Blood pressure increases
3. Muscle tension increases
4. G.S.R. decreases
5. Respiratory rate increases

6. Oxygen consumption increases

7. Spasm of arteries

8. S. Cortisol increases

9. S. Catecholamines increase

10. Blood sugar increases

11. Serum cholesterol increases

12. Acid in stomach increases

13. Blood clotting increases

14. Drying of saliva

15. Bowel and bladder tone decreases

Stress-related diseases

Modern science, till some years back, did not attribute stress to the creation of diseases. High blood pressure, heart disease, peptic ulcer are very common in highly placed executives and not so in a satisfied, moderately earning individual or a villager. This interesting fact can only be explained on the basis of severe stress that the former experiences.

In the last few decades a series of epidemiological studies and observations have proved that some very common diseases are a direct result of excessive stress. These are now grouped as psychosomatic diseases.

A List of the Common Diseases is as follows :

1. High blood pressure

2. Angina or chest pain

3. Heart attacks (myocardial infarction)

> Small stress reduction tip :
> Do not neglect family time.

4. Tension, headache

5. Migraine

6. Backache

7. Shoulder ache

8. Spondylosis

9. Palpitation

10. Allergies

11. Asthma

12. Chronic fatigue and lethargy

13. Anxiety state

14. Phobias

15. Insomnia

16. Depression

17. Irritable bowel syndrome (IBS)

18. Peptic ulcer

19. Pre-menstrual syndrome in females

Do you suffer from any of these? Be honest with yourself and try to identify and understand your problems and their proportions. This will help you to clearly define a solution for them.

Small stress reduction tip : Lunch should be away from the office.

Model of stress management

These values keep on changing slowly over the years in order to adjust with our changing environment. Any stagnation or fast change in the internal factors makes a person more susceptible to stress. These values keep on

Small stress reduction tip : Learn to delegate.

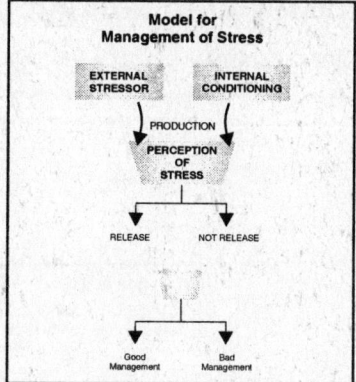

changing slowly over the years in order to adjust with our changing environment. Any stagnation or fast change in the internal factors makes a person more susceptible to stress.

How to cut down stress?

Stress reduction can be achieved first by identifying the stress symptoms and then following the next three steps:

1. Reduction in stress production

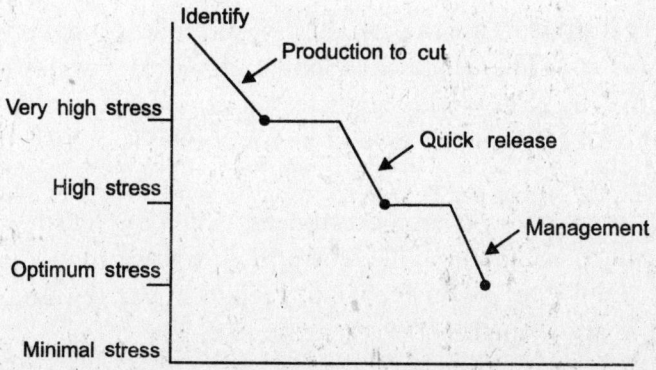

2. Releasing whatever stress is produced

3. Managing whatever stress is left

Small stress reduction tip : Develop a hobby that demands total concentration.

How is stress produced?

Production of Stress

Stress is the interaction between two major factors:

1. *External Stressors :* I would like to call it the stressor. I shall give a list of examples of possible stresses. Please identify them. An external stressor makes an almost equal contribution to stress. Even recognition of these is of great help in the management of stress.

2. *Internal Conditioning :* This is the result of our previous experiences, training, values and expectations. Our beliefs, hopes, attitudes and aspirations influence the internal factors.

External Stressors

External stressors are the causes or occurrences for the production of stress. These happen around us. If we react well to them, they may be good in reducing stress. If we know how to handle them better, we may be able to produce even happiness out of them.

External stressors are occurrences, which are mostly out of our control. Something like corruption, trains running late, a difficult boss, an aggressive family member, overcrowding, traffic jams are examples of external stressors.

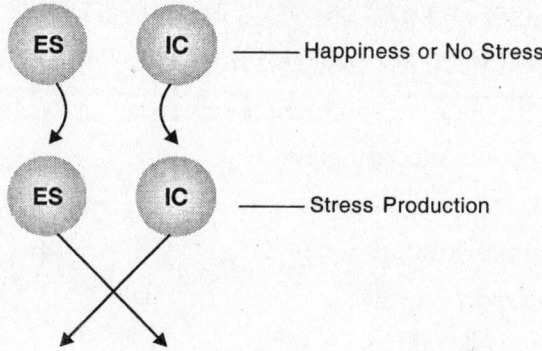

Happiness or No Stress

Stress Production

Examples of the External Stressors

Social and Family

1. High and unrealistic expectations
2. Difference in interests of wife/husband
3. Lack of communication with members
4. Recurrent financial problems
5. Different values and priorities
6. Different sleeping patterns
7. An ugly or a beautiful wife
8. Differences about work sharing
9. A talkative spouse
10. A rude spouse/member
11. Illness of a family member
12. Frequent guests
13. Unfaithfulness
14. Relatives with unreasonable expectations
15. Difficult neighbours

Occupation

1. Change little mores requiring new skills
2. Boss with abrasive communication style
3. Incompetent subordinates
4. Uncooperative colleagues
5. Poor administration
6. Bureaucracy
7. Numerous deadlines
8. Socialising during work
9. Lack of control over work environment
10. Lack of feedback from the top or bottom
11. Inadequate rewards
12. Time and work overload
13. Unclear authority
14. Long working hours
15. No holidays

Political

1. Unsteady political scenario
2. Corrupt ministers/members of parliament
3. Corrupt or non co-operative bureaucrats
4. Lack of leadership
5. Dictatorship
6. Strikes
7. International tension
8. Unfulfilled promises
9. Wrong media coverage
10. Industrial policy

11. Politicizing of religion
12. Repeated demonstrations/violence
13. Incompetent ministers
14. Criminals in politics
15. Unfair elections

Ecology

1. Increasing pollution
2. Deforestation
3. Urban crowding
4. Unplanned cities and towns
5. Adulteration of food
6. Loss of natural resources
7. Water pollution
8. Over industrialization
9. Radiation hazard
10. Noise pollution
11. Industrial accidents
12. Nuclear arms race
13. Ozone layer depletion
14. Extinction of rare animals
15. Green house effect

Physical and Psychological

1. Extreme hot or cold atmosphere
2. Dress, too tight or loose
3. Noisy surroundings at work/home
4. Uncomfortable chairs

5. Poor lighting and ventilation
6. Continuous bending, standing
7. Excessive eye strain
8. Lack of cleanliness
9. Lack of safety regulations
10. Sarcastic remarks
11. Politics in office
12. Hostile atmosphere
13. Isolated atmosphere
14. Overcrowded environment
15. People who create problems

Moral Values and Social Changes

1. Generation gap
2. Lack of morality
3. Class discrimination
4. Permissiveness/openness
5. Human rights violation
6. Violence
7. Movies, TV, books giving wrong messages
8. Social isolation
9. Housing shortage
10. Disharmony with the neighbours
11. Changed feelings about parents and teachers
12. Unfair trade or practices
13. Undependable friends and relatives
14. Social outcasts
15. Plight of sick, poor or old

Economic

1. Inflation
2. Slow economic growth
3. Water crisis
4. Power shortage
5. Union power
6. Reduced productivity
7. Export-import gap
8. Rich-poor gap
9. Excessive price of land and housing
10. Rising interest rates
11. Lack of cash flow
12. Bureaucracy in financial institutions
13. Cut in public expenditure
14. Over population and competitions for jobs
15. Fast changing technology

> Those who flow as life flows, know they need no other force. They feel no wear, they feel no tear, they need no mending, no repair.
> — LAO-TZU, THE WAY OF LIFE

What to do about external stressors?

As I have already explained, external stressors are to be handled with utmost care. If you understand them well, categorise them properly, looking at the practical aspects of life and deal with them appropriately, external stressors can be managed very well to your advantage. They cannot only cut down the stress production but can also make you happy.

Let us see what are the ways to deal with them:

> God give me strength to change the things I can, the tolerance to bear the things I cannot and the wisdom to know the difference.

1. Identify
2. Modify
3. Avoid
4. Accept
5. Fight
6. Be indifferent
7. Do not interpret negatively

If I try to describe these and other aspects of stress management completely, I may need to have another two hundred pages. This is probably going to be my next book. Here, I am just trying to discuss the salient points.

Identify

Identification is probably half the solution. If I can identify that trains run late because of the mis-management of the entire Indian railways, the stress because of trains arriving late is half solved. The rains, summer and winter fail to generate any stress, if we just understand the cyclic of nature for them. There is a difficult boss you are working with, just identify, and the stress is reduced. The first and the foremost thing is to identify the stressor.

Modify

There are external stressors which can be modified to a great extent. If there is a bulb of 25 watts in a toilet and the toilet looks dirty, then putting a bright tubelight can solve the uneasiness. Similarly, if you are getting late for office everyday, and you understand that you waste a lot of time procrastinating on the bed, or sleeping late, you can easily modify this.

> Small stress reduction tip : While you delegate, select a proper person and explain/train.

Avoid

Some external stressors are better to be avoided. It may be a difficult relative or neighbour, it is better to avoid them. They cannot be modified; so it will be better to pass them off and keep minimum contact. If a particular bank's services do not improve, we can always avoid that inefficient banking system and look for a more efficient one. Similarly if someone speaks or talks a lot in foul language and you do not like it, avoidance is the best formula then.

Accept

Many external stressors like corruption in society, a difficult father or a perfectionist wife, a selfish brother, situations which cannot be changed are best to be accepted. Many customs in society, and fashions that you do not like also fall in the same category. You have to decide what you want.

Fight

There are situations where something can neither be accepted nor avoided. In such cases, it is better to fight back. Someone has borrowed some five lac rupees and refuses to return it, the ideal way would be to fight. There are few such situations, where fighting back may be the best option. But remember such situations should be rare. Fighting should be allowed when no other option is left. Some people who pick up at least one fight everyday are called Type-A and are much more stressed.

Be Indifferent

Much of the external stressors which have no relevance to the basic needs of life are to be overlooked. This reduces stress

> Your health is bound to be affected if day after day you say the opposite of what you feel.
> — BORIS PASTERMNAK

which has no major importance in life. Political statements, incidents of terrorism, police cases reported in newspapers, winning of football teams, corruption cases against politicians are items in this category. Some people have a habit of putting their nose where not required. This causes unnecessary stress.

Do not Interpret Negatively

In this world there are many situations which we can never imagine or have come across in the past. Many external stressors were previously unknown. A human being has a tendency to reject things which are unknown to him. This often causes stress, because everyday new things happen. We should accept or reject a new thing after analysing and learning more about it.

Small stress reduction tip : Expect the best from people and give them the benefit of doubt.

Internal conditioning or mindsets

Internal Conditioning

Internal conditioning is the second item in the production of stress. It can also be called the mindset for better understanding. A newborn does not have any mindset. So he does not have objections to many of the happenings. The gradual building up of internal conditioning makes people happy or unhappy.

If I am a vegetarian by internal conditioning then serving of non-vegetarian food will produce stress. On the other hand, a non-vegetarian will have no stress. The difference is because of internal conditioning. The external stressors can be interpreted according to the internal conditioning to mindset — to produce or not to produce stress.

> *Whenever two good people fight over principles they are both right.*
> — ESCHENBACH

Let us see, what is internal conditioning and how does it develop in the following pages.

- ❑ Your likes, dislikes, beliefs and views
- ❑ Your value system and morality
- ❑ Your priorities
- ❑ Your social expectations
- ❑ Your disposition towards perfection and responsibilities
- ❑ Your training in communication
- ❑ Your materialistic expectations
- ❑ Your disposition for the protection of your ego

Factors Influencing Internal Conditioning

- ❑ Prevailing social structure
- ❑ Your mother
- ❑ Your family
- ❑ Your school and education
- ❑ People you have grown up with
- ❑ Your religion, spiritual training
- ❑ Your physical build-up
- ❑ Media : TV, books, movies, radio, newspaper
- ❑ Availability of financial resources, supports
- ❑ Personal experiences: fights, gains, losses, happiness, disappointments

How to change the mindset or internal conditioning?

There are only two options to cut down the stress production. One is to deal with the external stressors appropriately and the second is to change the internal conditioning as that is a more practical thing to do. Many people wonder whether it is possible to change the mindset.

According to SAAOL it is definitely possible and can be done by everyone. Our internal conditioning or mindsets change with time. Till sometime ago someone was a friend, today he may become an enemy. Internal conditionings do change. I might not have liked noodles till two years back, but today I may find them tasty. It is all internal conditioning.

When we talk about changing of internal conditioning, one must note that once it is understood, it becomes much easier to change. If one appreciates the reasons, it is also easy to change. I offer three reasons to change the internal conditionings.

1. Change with society
2. Understand *Anekant*
3. Society is based on give-and-take

Change with Society

Fashions are changing everyday, society is changing, dresses and behaviours have changed over the years. If you do not change your mindset or internal conditionings accordingly, you are liable to be confronted with the changed situations.

The sons previously (say 20 years back) used to touch their fathers' feet every morning, students used to do the same for their teachers, but now, if you expect the same, you will be greatly disappointed and stressed. This is called generation gap. The new group, the new ideas do not match because the old refuse to change. New cannot be held back. Now there are only two possibilities left — let them stay separately or let the old generation appreciate new ideas. The second possibility is the only viable possibility, new ideas have to enter your mindset everyday.

One does not require to change completely in one day. But you should keep an open mind. A few new ideas everyday will be good enough.

Understand *Anekant*

Anekant is a word from Jain philosophy which stands for 'theory of multiple view-points'. *Anekant* says that everyone would behave or think in his own way and he has a right to do so. 'Anek' means more than one. In other words, it means, more than one opinion about a single event or object.

If the father wants to do something in one way, the son may want it done in a different way. According to *Anekant*, both are right from their points of view. Their opinions will originate from their internal conditioning or mindsets. Both have the right to think in their own way.

If one of the family members wants the cleaning of the house to be done very thoroughly, the other person can also plan not to do so. One is very conscious about cleaning and the other feels that there are more constructive things to be done rather than cleaning. According to *Anekant* both are correct.

If you appreciate the theory of *Anekant*, you can change your internal conditioning easily. You will be able to understand others more clearly and analyse their ways of thinking. You will also be able to accept others' point of view. If not acceptable, at least you will be able to understand them. The production of stress will definitely be reduced. *Anekant* is the greatest theory in stress management.

Society is Based on Give and Take

The third way to modify the production of stress is 'give and take'. If two people with different ideas want to stay together, work together, there will be differences in their views, opinions.

No two persons can think alike. This leads to the need of compromise of 'give and take'.

Both have to give up some of their needs or ideas in order to fulfil the needs or ideas of the other. This is the rule of a healthy society. Sacrifice is a must. If both are adamant in their views then the group would break up soon. In relationships, if there are disputes everyday and both are adamant in their views, the relationship will produce plenty of stress or would break.

It is necessary that all the members of the society or group should understand this theory. This is one of the reasons we include the spouses in our SAAOL Heart Program training. If I could include the other family members too, it would be wonderful.

Small stress reduction tip : Keep your sense of humour.

The theory of *Anekant:* best way to manage stress

Theory of Multiple Viewpoints *(Anekant)*

Anekant, or the theory of multiple, different viewpoints stresses upon the fact that a single event is bound to be analyzed differently by separate individuals. This depends upon one's training, moral values, priorities and so on. Every person has his own thinking and right to express his views. By following *Anekant* one avoids many conflicts and helps oneself to perceive the different opinions of others.

Story of an Elephant and Three Blind Persons

There were three blind persons who were asked to describe an elephant after touching it.

The first one said that the elephant was like a pillar — the person reached the legs only and commented. The second one said it is like a rope by feeling the tail. The third person said it was like a hand fan as he touched the elephant's ear.

Anekant says that everyone with their own understanding, experience and feelings can express different opinions about the same thing. The story beautifully depicts the meaning of *Anekant*.

Anyone who maintains absolute standards of good or evil is dangerous. As dangerous as a maniac with a loaded revolver. In fact, the person who maintains absolute standards of good and evil usually is a maniac with a revolver.

— Tom Robbins

The art of communication: how to talk without stress

Communication Skill

Most of the stresses or fights occur because of bad ways of talking i.e. lack of knowledge about the art of communication. If you know how to communicate you will never have a fight. Dr. Ornish uses the communication skill very well and I have learnt it from him.

The art of talking or communicating is very important for avoiding stress for an executive, official or a family man. Half of our social stresses are due to bad skills of communication. Some tips about this aspect are as follows :

1. Listen when the other person talks. Everyone wants to be heard.

2. Do not criticize directly. Don't insult. Only express your feelings.

3. Speak softly but come to the point.
4. Use your understanding of non-verbal communication before you start.
5. For a regular and smooth communication bring down the tone of communication.

Since our hearts can speak a language that no one hears or sees and, therefore, cannot understand we can get sick at heart.

— James J. Lynch

How to handle anger

When You are Angry

1. Do not act in haste. Let your anger simmer down.
2. Think of the positive side of criticism.
3. Use anger creatively, perform some other jobs which need only your participation e.g. clear a pending account work or read a tax chapter.
4. Talk to your close associates or friends.
5. Learn the art of forgiveness

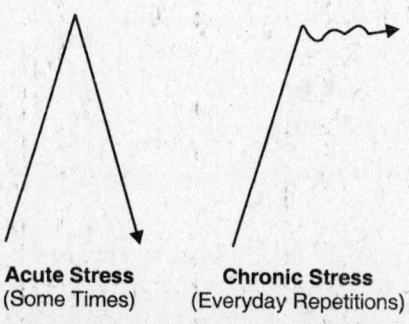

Acute Stress   Chronic Stress
(Some Times)   (Everyday Repetitions)

Stress can be acute or chronic. Acute stress is when you are suddenly angry. Chronic stress means the stress coming everyday from the same event.

Anger and intolerance are the twin enemies of correct understanding.

— M GANDHI

How to solve chronic stress?

1. Try to reach the root cause of the problem. Suggest an honest answer or solution.
2. Train yourself to understand non-verbal communication, half of what one talks gets reflected non-verbally.
3. Change your own dialogue once you know you are wrong.
4. Be persistent in small promises.
5. Assertive social conversation, assert your need and do not suffer because of this.
6. Understand your critic.
7. Respond to your critic appropriately.
8. Make workable compromises.
9. Change expectation to intention.
10. Positive thinking.

Small stress reduction tip : Learn to accept limitations in yourself.

Time management

There are 24 hours in a day. All of us, starting from the President of India to the topmost industrialist or a beggar manage our own work in the same time frame. How best can you complete all your duties or responsibilities depends on your time management skills. You must plan. Best is to decide a long term plan and then from time to time, work out a small time schedule.

Sleep should ideally be of 6 to 7 hours duration. Keep at least 1-2 hours for your family on a week day and try to spend major part of the holidays with the family. Daily chores should take about 2-3 hours (bathing, dressing, breakfast etc.). Rest of the time is for work.

Now, set your priorities and divide your time. If you feel your duties are difficult to manage within a given time span, then consider delegating some duties to your junior or refuse the job. Try to stick to your daily routine and relax on holidays. If you analyse, many of us do not actually spend time in actual working but waste it.

A List of Time Wasters is Provided Below

1. Telephone interruptions
2. Meetings
3. Visitors
4. Socializing
5. Lack of information
6. Excessive paper work
7. Communication breakdown
8. Lack of policies, procedures and coordinations
9. Lack of competent personnel
10. Red tape
11. Procrastination
12. Failure to delegate
13. Unclear objectives

14. Failure to set priorities
15. Crisis management
16. Poor scheduling
17. Lack of self discipline
18. Attempting to do too much at one time
19. Lack of relevant skills.

Early to bed and early to rise, makes a man healthy, wealthy and wise.

— FRANKLIN

Meditation and *Kayotsarg*

One of the best ways to manage stress is the practice of meditation. In our SAAOL camps I use *Preksha* meditation — one of the finest ways to meditate. Preksha means 'to see deeply' or 'to perceive deeply'. You just have to observe intensely the focus of the meditation, be it an organ or an imaginary point or an idea. *Preksha* meditation was developed by the well known saint and scholar Acharya Mahaprajna and Late Acharya Shree Tulsi. Both are well known Jain gurus.

I have only modified the meditation to suit my patients. The heart has been made the main focus of the meditation that I use. For stress management, practice of meditation for a minimum of fifteen minutes everyday is highly recommended.

Kayotsarg means relaxation. This is an advanced way of relaxing the body and mind. It can be termed as progressive relaxation and is a very powerful tool to release stress. I will describe it in more detail in the chapter on Yoga. I would be happy if my patients spend about fifteen minutes a day on *Kayotsarg*. I have developed some audio cassettes, keeping this in mind, which are now available at my centres.

Stress may not only adversely alter blood vessels but also elevate the cholesterol level in the blood. A number of studies have shown that blood cholesterol can be reduced by meditation.

— VOLTAIRE

Belief in God — an important tool for stress management

I advise that belief in God or the Almighty is a very important way a to cut down stress. Love, sacrifice and devotion that are attached to praying to God are exceptional. They not only calm the mind but also imbibe a lot of humbleness in the human mind. Only the human mind can understand God. In the western countries, the concept of God is less popular, but it is a must here.

God does not limit Himself to any sect or to any community. He is above caste. I strongly discourage the introduction of any particular God in the SAAOL concept. Everyone can choose his God (there are more than 1000 names in India for God.) I would be satisfied with one only.

I distribute some bhajan cassettes to develop devotion for God and recommend my patients to hear the songs which can change them completely. The bhajan cassettes can be played when you do yogasana.

Small stress reduction tip : Know what is going on — don't shut of your eyes.

Role of meditation and pranayama in stress management

Understanding stresses, analysing their production, tips to solve them have no doubt a very important role in stress management, but something will still be missing if we do not speak of meditation or pranayama. These two branches of yoga are probably the two most important tools to control stress or tension. Meditation is calming of the mind — one has to practice it for at least fifteen minutes every day to keep one's mind under control. Meditation produces Alpha waves in the brain and leads to a stabilising effect on our Limbic brain (Limbic system in the human brain is responsible for emotions like anger, fear, fury, and irrational behaviour). Without meditation no one can control their emotions. One must remember meditation is more of a practical experience and not a theoretical proposition. One has to do it properly to feel the difference. A book can only give you an idea, but it cannot give you the feeling. I have talked about meditation in more detail in the next chapter on Yoga.

Pranayama — on the other hand — is a practice of slow and long breathing and is immensely beneficial for managing stresses. I advise people to practice Nadi-sodhan pranayama (Anulom Vilom Pranayama) for five to ten minutes to cut down tension. Pranayama leads to more power to the rational mind or cerebral cortex of the brain. People who practice Pranayama become more rational and can understand others better.

Developing moral values (*Anuvrat*)

Erosion of moral values is one of the major causes of the social, cultural and behavioural decay in modern times. Everybody knows about this but somehow seems to be unconcerned. In order to develop a good personality we must follow the principles of *Anuvrat* which believes in the following:

1. Existence of others
2. Unity of mankind
3. Communal harmony

4. Non-violence
5. Limitation of acquisition and consumption
6. Integrity in behaviour
7. Purity of means
8. Fearlessness and truthfulness

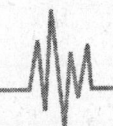

Section 9

Food and Coronary Heart Disease

Contents

The way to a man's heart is through his stomach.

— Sorah Payson Parton

The discovery of a new dish does more for human happiness than the discovery of a new star.

— BRILLAT SAVARIN

Introduction

Heart disease, the most common killer disease, is affected by the kind of food one eats. In my experience wrong food contributes to, on an average, 30% of the causes of heart disease.

If we consider the human body as a machine then the fuel is food. As a car, scooter, train or aeroplane uses fuel in the form of petrol or diesel, our body uses food as the fuel for running the machine. Without this fuel the body cannot work. This fuel in the form of food is needed by everyone and thus eating forms a very important part of our lives.

Some of us work hard to earn this fuel. Others get more than adequate quantity. But the body needs fuel according to its use, in the form of physical activity or exercise. If you supply more it can store this fuel.

There are three kinds of food fuels that the body can use — carbohydrates, proteins and fats. All the food items that we eat have different proportions of these three items. Some have more carbohydrates like rice and wheat; some have more proteins like mutton and pulses and some are loaded with fat like butter and oils. Each of them can act as a fuel for the body.

Though the body can break any of these foods for fuel (energy or power) in the short run as an emergency, it is best to properly balance the three fuels for long term smooth running of the body. When born, the body is made in such a way that it will run for about hundred years and thus a balancing of these fuels is of utmost importance. Without this there will be defects in the body and when these reach a significant magnitude it results in diseases.

> If the doctors of today don't become dieticians the dieticians of tomorrow will become doctors.

Most people are unaware of these important aspects of food and eating; though it forms one of the most important aspects of our everyday life. Lack of knowledge in this respect sooner or later lands us in ill health.

The dieticians, who are supposed to be experts in these subjects, are either taken lightly or taken seriously only when the disease actually occurs. Even then, people follow their advice for a short while till the disease is controlled. Dieticians also do not give their patients the basic information and concepts. They advise them for a temporary period. This has led to non-education of the people, who become potential patients mainly due to lack of knowledge.

Medical doctors, on their part, find it below their dignity to talk about food and nutrition. These physicians generally consider their duty as only to intervene in an emergency. Once the emergency is tackled, they do not usually try to prevent the future possibility of another emergency because by then they are trying to solve somebody's else emergency.

The brunt of these happenings has been thus borne by the patients and apparently healthy people who are gradually going towards full fledged diseases.

The aim of writing this book is to make people aware of the actual fuel requirement of the body, to increase their knowledge about the composition of various kinds of food available, to advise them what to do and what not to do (with reasons) and to teach them how to cook the same with excellent taste. In this way they can put into practice what they have learnt in their practical life.

> Thirty percent of the products in the grocery store today could be thrown out and nobody would be any the worse.
>
> — Prof. D Marl Hegsted

A very important role in the formation of blockages in the coronary arteries is attributed to diet, the type of food we eat, the quantity of food we consume, and of course its direct relationship to the calculated calorie requirements for our daily routine.

Diet has a bifactoral relationship with coronary heart disease, as we will see later. Firstly, it is related to Coronary Heart Disease in terms of calories (energy) and secondly in terms of fat intake. This is quite simple to understand if think about total energy intake in terms of calories to the amount of energy that we spend everyday. For example; if the total amount of calories spent in our daily routine is 1600 kcal, we have the tendency of always eating much more than our daily requirements. We never consume less than what is actually required to perform our daily chores. The extra amount is stored in the form of fat, which also gets deposited not only in the body but also in the inner linings of the blood vessels. Over time cholesterol gradually increases giving rise to severe obstruction to blood flow through the vessels which in turn results in coronary artery disease.

It is an established fact that levels of cholesterol and triglycerides in our blood are directly correlated with our diet; that is to say the more food we consume rich in fats, our blood cholesterol level rises, and the faster is the cholesterol deposits formation in coronary blood vessels. Foods rich in animal fats such as egg yolk, mutton, milk (non-skimmed), fish, prawns, ghee, butter etc., foodstuff such as nuts and dry fruits are also responsible for the elevation of blood cholesterol levels. It is, thus, important to pay particular attention to diet in the management of coronary heart disease. If this aspect is neglected, the blockages in the blood vessels of the heart will continue to grow in size despite all our efforts to treat the disease medically or surgically.

For a properly integrated approach to treating coronary heart disease, it is essential to withhold and reduce cholesterol contents in our daily diets. The SAAOL Heart Program advocates a strict vegetarian diet where even milk is restricted to a minimum permissible limit. Animal fats and proteins, along with alcohol are absolutely forbidden. This implementation is mandatory not only to arrest the growth in the size of the blockage, but also to bring about a reduction in size — the ultimate phenomena of reversal, thus curing coronary heart disease permanently!

Before thirty, men seek disease, atfer thirty diseases seek men.

— A Proverb

What are calories — how many calories do we need or spend?

What are Calories?

As we measure money in rupees, weight in kilograms, energy is measured in calories. For any work we do, we need calories. If I talk for a minute, I need about 2 calories. If I run, I need about 10 calories in a minute. Even when we sleep our heart has to continue beating and we have to continue breathing. These functions need about half a calorie every minute.

What is Your Calorie Spending?

In a normal day most people (those not engaged in physical labour like porters or labourers) require about 1600 calories in a day. A labourer may require 3000 calories. If you don't do any work and only sleep throughout the day and night, you will probably require about 800 calories per day. I am giving you a chart of how many calories approximately we require when we do the usual activities.

Activity approximate per minute	Calories
Sleep	0.6 calories
Reading	1.4 calories
Eating	1.8 calories
Converse	1.8 calories
Writing	1.9 calories
Driving a car	2.1 calories
Standing	2.2 calories
Slow walking	3 to 4 calories
Casual walking	4 to 5 calories
Fast walking	6 to 8 calories
Jogging	7 to 9 calories
Running	10 to 12 calories

If you apply your mind a little more you will be able to estimate how many calories you spend while sewing, gossiping or playing badminton.

Someone who spends 1600 calories in a day, takes food in such a quantity that it will provide 1600 calories in a day, will have no excess or deficiency. It is like a bank account.

There are two kinds of failures; those who thought and never did and those who did and never thought.

Components of Food

All food items that we consume (by anybody all over the world) can be divided into seven scientifically named groups. These are called carbohydrates, proteins, fats, vitamins, minerals, fibres and water. No other item is available in any food, other than these seven. Our body requires all these for growth, maintenance and development. Without any of these, the body will not be able to survive, but excess intake can also cause damage. Therefore, we must know how much food for each of these is to be consumed for best health. We should also be aware of their functions. This is what we will discuss in this chapter.

Of course I do not want you to become doctors and dieticians, but I would like to provide adequate information, so that you can consciously decide about what you want to eat and what would be the best combination that you can choose.

Carbohydrates are foods which give you energy that you require for your daily activities. They sustain you throughout the day. Proteins are the building blocks of the body. They form the bulk of the muscles of the body. They are the main constituents of the wall of each cell of the body. They are also the major components of the nerves. Fats, the so-called oils and cholesterol — are also components of the cell wall, the nerve cells and the brain. Fats also form the energy storage of the body. Whenever there is excess energy supplied to the body (in the form of foods eaten throughout the day) they will get converted into fats and get stored inside the body. This is what leads to overweight and heart disease.

Vitamins are the protective food items which protect the skin, eyes, bones, nerves and the heart. Without adequate vitamins we are prone to many diseases like blindness, bleeding gums, weak bones and a degenerated brain. Vitamins are required in very small quantities.

Minerals like calcium, potassium, and sodium form the bones, give strength to the structure of the body, form a major part in haemoglobin and form the digestive enzymes, and help in breaking the food (metabolism). We get minerals through all common food items and juices.

Fibres are food items that cannot be utilised by the body but are essential in the metabolism of life. They help in curing by removing constipation, stopping the absorption of cholesterol and preventing cancer. Fibres are very important for reduction of weight and control of diabetes. Fruits, vegetables and sprouts are very rich in fibres.

Water does not have any energy (or calories) but is probably the most important part of our intake. No function of the body can be carried out without water right from chewing to digesting and absorbing food. Water is required for hundreds of functions of the body. Water forms more than 50% of blood, helps in excretion of toxins from the body through the kidneys, regulates temperature of the body and most importantly helps in carrying oxygen to all the parts of the body.

In this chapter we are going to discuss a lot more scientific information about food and for those who want more scientific data, the following pages will be very important.

At a Glance

Foods that provide energy	Foods that provide vitality	Helpful food
Carbohydrates Proteins Fats	Vitamins Minerals Water	Fibres

Information given in plenty can also confuse many common readers. I have tried not to give much information on chemicals structures, reactions that lead to production of energy, how they are absorbed and so on. I have put efforts to simplify scientific information and screen out the unwanted information.

Zero oil food

According to SAAOL, out of the 1600 calories that are required by the body approximately 65-70% should come from carbohydrates, 20-25% should come from proteins and the balance 10% should come from fats. Since this 10% of the calories coming from fats are equivalent to about 18 grams of fat, they can be met through the invisible sources of fat — such as rice, wheat, pulses and cereals. SAAOL recommends no oil (which is nothing but fat) in the food.

It is imperative that all the food eaten by the people with heart disease should have no visible oil in it, in order to bring about a reversal.

The common belief is that without oil as a cooking medium no good food can be prepared or cooked. Almost all households use oil (fat extract of many natural food items marketed by hundreds of oil companies) to prepare, cook and season spices, while cooking food. Some of the common names of these oils available in India are Saffola, Cornola, Dhara, Dalda, Sweekar, Sundrop, Gold winner, Sanola, Postman, Mastan, Palmoil, Sungold. Ghee which is another Indian fat used popularly as a cooking medium is derived from milk. The cooking methods described in this chapter do not use any oil. That is why it is called zero oil. One must remember that the use of these oils can be detrimental to our health as in the modern era we do not exercise or perform physical activity required to utilize these high calorie fatty items. We understand that some fat is necessary for our body and can be obtained from the invisible or hidden fat in the natural and so called non-fatty items. We also do not recommend any milk products or extracts like cheese, butter, cream or margarine as they also contain very high amount of oil.

Eat to live and not live to eat.

— A PROVERB

Will the food taste good?

In our camps organised for the heart patients during the last few years, we found that most of the worry about taste in the zero oil food items is from the misconception that without oil food cannot give a good taste.

Years of practice of cooking food using oil or ghee has almost wiped out our ideas about cooking good food without oil. We cannot even imagine such a situation. From generations Indian cooking has used one or the other fat. The conditioning has been so deep-rooted, that whenever I talked about zero oil food, people have shown disbelief. When I talk of good taste without oil, many ladies have questioned my experience with cooking.

I noticed during my practice that whenever I told my patients to eat food without oil or ghee they ate boiled food. Then they would complain about bland taste. They couldn't imagine eating boiled food for a long time.

Many of the housewives and experienced ladies then started cooking food with a little oil, after a strong advice from me against oils for heart patients. When I argue, they say it is impossible to season the spices, *masalas*, in India without oil.

Questioned by so many experienced people, a few years back I really started developing recipes without oil or ghee, because I understood that I could not give my patients these two items as they would increase the fats in the blood and lead to further deposits. The beginning was difficult. I asked myself why couldn't I season the *masalas* without oil, may be using only water. The answer came handy, cook it with water and see.

When I was conducting courses at the All India Institute of Medical Sciences I could not really do a lot of innovations in cooking. I used to advise the patients to eat fruits, boiled vegetables, dal (cooked pulses), khichadi (a combination of rice and different kinds of pulses). People complained, but would eat it as they were scared of heart attacks.

But after starting my private set-up, where I had a free hand, I started looking into other possibilities. We experimented along with the cooks at the resorts, where we were holding our camps, and with the help of our gifted dieticians and the idea of cooking things with water for seasoning and the results were wonderful. We prepared a number of items. Then there was no looking back. And now we have hundreds of recipes.

Talking about the taste, I must tell you the food items that SAAOL makes taste as good as any other oil-cooked foods. Our patients know it. The hotels where I conducted the courses cooked foods often much better than the usual. If you ask me why there is no difference in the taste, the answer will be that we use all the *masalas* which give the taste, the only difference being that we use water instead of oil to season those *masalas*.

So simple, is it not?

The kind of people who always go on about whether a thing is in good taste, invariably have a very bad taste.

— JEO ORTON

Vegetarian food vs non-vegetarian food

As a Jain, right from my childhood, I was taught that vegetarianism is the only choice we have, because Jains are forbidden non-vegetarian food. Later, I realized, as a medical doctor that vegetarianism is also scientifically advantageous.

When I devised food for preventing or curing heart disease, I minutely analyzed the advantages and disadvantages of both kinds of foods. I could find that one of the major contributors of coronary disease has been meats and the yellow of egg. All kinds of meats are rich sources of cholesterol (which get deposited inside the arteries) and triglycerides (fats). They have very little fibres. Though chicken and fish are better, but they too can lead to aggravation of heart disease. A lot of oil and ghee is also used to cook these meat preparations.

Another factor that aggravated my feelings against meat is probably the secretion of some chemicals called adrenaline and adrenaline-like substances inside these animals when they are killed to harvest the meat. Man basically is a vegetarian animal — consider the gut or the teeth or the health — vegetarianism is the hallmark of human beings. Most of the flesh eaters are more prone to be short tempered and aggressive — may be the chemicals, secreted just before the death of the animal which contributed to the meat, are responsible for the same.

On the other hand vegetarian food has a variety of salads and cereals, legumes which offer better health. Vitamins, minerals and antioxidants are plenty in vegetarian food. Fruits are rich in minerals, trace materials, carotenes, flavonoids which are always healthy. The fibres present in vegetarian food are plenty thereby preventing heart disease, overweight and cancer.

The only non-vegetarian item I allow is probably the white of an egg. There is no fat in it and this can be scientifically allowed to heart patients. Inclusion of these three items, in the book indicates that I still prefer science above my religious belief.

Now, vegetarianism has taken a lead over non-vegetarianism. People in the west have returned to vegetarianism after being non-vegetarians. We Indians who have a tradition of vegetarianism, supported by religion, are still going, unfortunately, towards non-vegetarianism. I hope good sense would prevail soon!

What is food for one man is bitter poison to others.

— LUCRETIUS

Food and enjoyment

When we eat food, whether it leads to pleasure or unhappiness, depends on our social upbringing, exposure to different food items in the past and so on. This behaviour I call as 'Internal Conditioning'. This psychological factor determines whether one would like or dislike the food.

When I stayed in the hostel in my student days I used to have food which had no taste, the *chapatis* were hard and thick having such a bad look but I used to love them. Whenever any of my family members visited me they would wonder how I could consume such tasteless food. It was all due to internal conditioning.

For someone who eats meat or fish it is impossible to think of a meal without non-vegetarian food, as he is conditioned to it. But once he becomes a vegetarian, he will hate non-vegetarian food and wonder how he consumed it in the past. It is all a matter of internal conditioning.

When I moved to Delhi, I did not like Chinese food like chowmein and noodles. But going to Chinese restaurants regularly changed me. I enjoy these two items now. Apply this to yourself — you'll find you have done similar things in the past.

After I had started SAAOL, a non-vegetarian patient visited me. He asked, "Doctor you don't eat non-veg food?" I said, "No." He said, "Fifty percent of your enjoyment in life is gone." I asked, "Next." He asked, "Alcohol?" I said, "No." He said, "75% of life's enjoyment is gone." I asked what else? He enquired whether I smoked or took tea or coffee to which I replied in the negative. His ultimate opinion was: "You should commit suicide." Because he thought no pleasure was left in my life.

> An ass is beautiful to an ass and a pig is beautiful to a pig.
> — JOHN RAY

But I must tell you I enjoy my food better than many around me. It is a matter of understanding and internal conditioning.

Enjoyment of food depends on your habits and how thoroughly you have conditioned yourself. Once I asked a person to write down all the things he loved or things that gave happiness to him. There were more than one hundred items on the list. I just cut non-vegetarian food and two more items which were fried. He was still left with scores of items. It included his walks, his wife and children, his car, his work, his office, his friends, TV, movies and music !

One half of the world cannot understand the pleasures of the other.

— *Jane Austen*

Carbohydrates

Carbohydrates supply energy and allow proteins to be used for tissue building and repair. In the reversal diet, almost 70% of the energy required by the body is provided by carbohydrates. The energy value of 1 g of carbohydrate is 4 kcal.

Composition

Carbohydrates contain carbon, hydrogen and oxygen. Some carbohydrates are relatively small molecules. Others are larger and more complex and consist of a few or more molecules linked in chains. The members of simplest class having single unit are monosaccharide. Glucose is an example of this class. The disaccharide contains two sugars — cane/beet sugar (sucrose) and milk (lactose) are members of this class. Carbohydrates made of long chains of sugars are polysaccharide e.g. being starch, glycogen, cellulose, plant gums and mucilages.

Functions

The main function of carbohydrates is to provide energy. They are a quick source of energy and also aid in the utilization of body fats and exert a sparing effect on proteins.

Food Sources

Carbohydrates are Synthesized by Plants

Sugar, cereal grains, legumes and dried fruits are the richest source of carbohydrates. White sugar is the richest. Cereals, grains, legumes and dried fruits vary in their carbohydrate contents. Some processed foods like noodles, dried non-fat milk, solids, jams, jellies, breads and candies contain appreciable quantities.

Fresh fruits and vegables are considered low in carbohydrates but bananas, dates, white potatoes and sweet potatoes are its rich sources.

Deficiency

If less than the requirement of carbohydrates are consumed, the body first burns its own fat and then its tissue protein for energy. To prevent this the daily requirement should be met regularly.

Proteins

Protein is the most abundant component of the body next to water. 1g of this nutrient provides 4 kcal of energy. A major portion of the proteins is located in the muscle tissues, the remainder is widely distributed in the blood, other soft tissues, bones and teeth. Proteins are present in all living tissues, both plants and animals.

Proteins are built from 23 or more simpler compounds called amino acids, often called 'building stones'. Of 23 or more amino acids present in plants and animals, some can be synthesized in sufficient quantities in the body. Eight amino acids are essential for maintenance and cannot be synthesized in the body. These have to be supplied by food and are called essential amino acids.

The quality of protein depends on the kind and amount of essential amino present in that food. e.g. cereals are low in lysine and pulses contain a small amount of methionine. But cereals and pulses are normally consumed together with other foods such as vegetables, curd, etc., so deficiency of one is supplemented by the other food.

Functions of Proteins

1. Building new tissues in growth stages of life, from conception upto adulthood and after injury.
2. Maintenance of tissues already built and replacement of routine losses.
3. As regulatory substances for internal water and acid-base balance.
4. As precursors for enzymes, antibodies, some hormones and vitamin B.
5. For milk formation.
6. For energy.

Food Sources

Plants are the primary source of proteins because they can synthesize proteins by combining nitrogen and water from soil, and CO_2 from air.

Although proteins are widely distributed in nature, a few foods provide them in highly concentrated form. Non-vegetarian and milk products (not recommended for reversal diet) are its primary sources. Cereals, grains, dals and legumes rank second and fruits and vegetables are low protein foods. Sugar, syrups, pure fats and oils contain no proteins.

Deficiency

Deficiency of proteins in diet results in stunted growth. If limitation is severe and prolonged, the protein content of blood may be reduced to below normal.

Fats

Fats are concentrated sources of energy in our diets. The reversal diet allows 10% of the total energy from fats. 1 g of the nutrient provides 9 kcal. The chemical term for a fat is 'Triglyceride'.

Composition

Fats are composed of carbon, hydrogen and oxygen. If the substance is a liquid, at 20^0 it is oil and if solid at room temperature, it is called fat. There are four parts of every fat molecule. The core of molecule is glycerol. The fatty acid is attached to each of the 3 carbon units of glycerol molecule.

The types of fats depend on saturation/unsaturation of fatty acids.

Certain fatty acids contain as many hydrogen atoms as the carbon chain can hold; these are called 'saturated'. There are others that have only one 'double bond' and are referred to as 'mono-unsaturated. A third group may have 2, 3, 4 or more 'double bonds' and is called 'polyunsaturated'.

Sources

The richest sources of fats in the diet are vegetable oils like corn oil, groundnut oil, olive oil, sesame seed oil, mustard oil, sunflower oil, coconut oil and animal fats like butter and ghee. Nuts are the highest contributors of fat. Meat, poultry and fish vary in their fat contents. All cheeses except cottage cheese (depending on the milk source) contain appreciable amounts of fat. The fat in egg is only concentrated in the yolk. Products like potato chips, cakes, pastries, cookies and candy bars also contain appreciable amount of fats. Most fruits and vegetables contain very little fats but avocado and coconut contain 20% fat.

Functions
1. Richest and concentrated source of energy.
2. They carry fat soluble vitamins (A, D, E, K) into the body and help in absorption of these vitamins which are necessary for growth in the young and maintenance of a healthy skin.
3. Since it is a bad conductor of heat, a layer beneath the skin helps to conserve body heat.
4. Acts as a cushion for the vital organs.
5. Increases palatability and satiety value of the food.

Deficiency or Excess
When the diet is deficient in fats or carbohydrates, the body tends to burn its own fat for energy. Continued deprivation of energy due to insufficiency of fat and carbohydrates in diet may lead to protein being used for energy. Therefore adequate amounts should be consumed.

In case there is an excess of fat it may result in:
1. Retardation in digestion and create body discomfort.
2. Excess fat storage and extra burden on the heart and other organs.

Minerals

Minerals are referred to as inorganic or ash constituents. In the body minerals provided in food remain after the organic compounds, of which they are a part, have been oxidized. About 4-6% of body weight is made of mineral elements. These minerals are nothing but elements like sodium, potassium, magnesium, calcium, manganese, iron, zinc, chlorine and their salts. Most of the minerals are present in natural fruits, vegetables and their juices. The largest concentration of minerals are found in the bones and teeth. Minerals are also found in soft tissues and in the blood and other body fluids.

Some of the functions of minerals are:
1. Maintenance of an acid-base balance
2. Control of water balance
3. Contraction of muscles
4. Normal response of nerves to physiological stimulation
5. Clotting of blood

Water: a very important component of food

Water

Water is an essential nutrient, yet one which is overlooked when talking of nutrient needs of the body. Approximately 55-70% of the total body weight is made of water. Actually it is possible to survive a longer time without food but not without water. The requirement depends on factors like environmental temperature, humidity, occupation and diet. In general, around 1.5-2 ltrs. of water per day is enough (apart from water obtained through food which one may eat).

Functions
Water is used in the body in a variety of ways.

i) as a building material in the construction of cells.

ii) as a solvent for normal functioning of the body cells i.e. the nutrients which are carried to the cells and waste products of metabolism are removed.

iii) as a lubricant in the joints and between internal organs.

iv) as a body temperature regulator and aids in the removal of heat from the body.

Sources

Water for the body comes from the fluids of the diet, the solid foods of the diet and the water produced by the metabolism of energy nutrients within tissues. Water contents of food vary widely, with most foods in an average diet containing more than 70% moisture e.g. green beans contains 92% water, while milk contains 87%.

Effect of Deficiency

The body normally maintains a water balance i.e. the amount of water ingested is equal to water excreted or lost.

Water is lost from the body through kidneys (urine), skin (perspiration), lungs (exhaled air), intestinal canal (faeces) and eyes (tears). The loss of water is influenced by the individual's physical activity, environmental temperature, due to diarrhoea, vomiting, protracted fever, etc. The severity may result in dehydration when the outflow of water exceeds the intake. Dehydration can be severe and calls for medical attention too. So this can be easily overcome by taking water, salt or special attention to water with minerals.

Fibres in food

Fibre is an important component in a healthy diet. This basically comes from plant based foods like cellulose, hemicellulose and pectins which are components of the skins of fruits. Coverings of seeds and structural parts of plants are also referred to as fibres. There are two types of dietary fibres — soluble and insoluble. Fibrous foods are filled with fewer calories. They also add roughage to the diet which in turn aids digestion and elimination. Since these are parts of plants that cannot be broken down in the intestines by human enzymes, so they can't be absorbed.

Soluble fibres can lower total blood cholesterol and LDL cholesterol. The mechanism is as yet unconfirmed but it is believed that people who eat more soluble fibres may eat less food which are high in saturated fats. Soluble fibres also slow down the movement of food through the small intestines.

Insoluble fibres themselves do not lower total blood cholesterol but they do fill up and contribute to proper bowel function. They also speed up the movement of food through the intestines and promote regularity. Cellulose, hemicellulose and pectins are insoluble fibres.

Dietary fibre has also been considered important for preventing constipation. The benefits of fibres for lowering cholesterol explain why heart disease is less frequently caused in people on a high fibre diet. Dietary fibre also helps in regulating blood sugar and has a favourable effect on blood pressure. Studies have been done, where fibres have shown protection against cancer especially of the colon and rectum.

Switching over to a high fibre diet from a low one should be done gradually so as to avoid diarrhoea, gas and other types of stomach and intestinal disorders.

What the processed-food-industry does to a grain of wheat is awesome. Basically they take out everything that is good for you and leave an absolutely bland, easily digestible white powder.

— RICHARD WATSON

The exact amount of fibres required by the human body cannot be accurately stated. This amount varies from 100 mg/ to 5 6 gm per day. But an average mixed diet consisting of raw vegetables, fresh fruits with skins, cooked vegetables and fruits will usually provide sufficient fibre. This quantity can be increased by use of some whole grains or whole wheat bread.

Food Sources

Soluble	Insoluble
Oat bran, rolled oats, broccoli, brussel sprouts, grapefruit, apples	Whole wheat bread, cereals, cabbage, carrots, turnips, cauliflower, asparagus, peas, kidney beans, wheat bran

Antioxidants in food

There is a group of supernutrients that are currently attracting the attention of medical and scientific researchers. In essence, these are precursors to vitamin A (called beta-carotene), vitamin C and vitamin E. Together, these nutrients form a powerful alliance which can help to protect the body from many diseases and also forestall the ageing process.

These vitamins are present in many types of food and occur naturally in fruits and vegetables which we can consume in plenty, especially when they are in season, whereas taking of drugs in comparison is fraught with side-effects and they are no match for natural nutrients. In fact, extensive research is being carried out in this direction supported by the WHO and other Food and Agriculture Ministries.

There have been numerous studies into extraordinary powers of beta-carotene, vitamin C and vitamin E. Studies have revealed that lung cancer, angina and other heart diseases are much less evident and longevity is established by a liberal intake of A, C and E vitamins.

Use of oxygen derived from food to fuel body processes is remarkable. Oxygen is moved around the body by red-coloured particles of haemoglobin that contain iron. Oxygen is taken in the bloodstream to feed living cells. This process is called oxidation. However, oxygen also creates free radicals, which cause problems when they are in excess.

Free radicals are the by-products of oxidation. When the body uses oxygen, it burns food to make energy. It also burns germs and toxic substances such as ozone and carbon monoxide. In the process free radicals are also produced. These radicals damage cell membranes, disturb chromosomes and genetic material and destroy valuable enzymes, causing a chain reaction of damage throughout the body. Thus, free radicals are a major cause of at least 50 per cent of diseases such as coronary heart disease, lung disease, certain cancers, cataracts, rheumatoid arthritis, Parkinson's disease and the ageing process.

There are two ways in which we can reduce the damage caused by free radicals. First, we should avoid substances and activities that encourage production of free radicals like cigarettes, pollution and ultraviolet radiation from the sun. The second step is to ensure that we consume plenty of antioxidants in our daily diet by relying on A,C,E vitamins.

Although A, C, E vitamins help combat effects of free radical damage, air pollution also reduces supply of these vital nutrients.

The end of man is knowledge, but there is one thing he can't know. He can't know whether knowledge will save him or kill him. He will be killed, all right, but he can't know whether he is killed because of the knowledge which he has got or because of the knowledge which he hasn't got and which, if he had it, would save him.

— ROBERT PENN WARREN

Studies have established that city dwellers who breathe polluted air have lower levels of antioxidants. This leaves the body short-changed and dangerously low in supplies of A, C, E vitamins. When this happens, free radicals take over and oxidative stress occurs.

The concept of antioxidants is relatively new. Medical science has propagated immense benefits of vitamins and the scientists have been striving hard to prove the authenticity of these magic substances.

Antioxidants are a powerful group of nutrients which protect the body from many diseases and also forestall the ageing process. They comprise B-carotene (vitamin A), vitamin C and vitamin E. These antioxidants help in combating the effects of free radical damage.

Antioxidants unravel a whole new avenue of treating a wide variety of pathological conditions such as:

i) Cardiovascular disease — CHD, high blood pressure

ii) Cerebrovascular disease — stroke

iii) Metabolic diseases — diabetes mellitus

iv) Neurological disease — Alzheimer's disease, epilepsy

v) Degenerative diseases — cataract, arthritis, ageing

vi) Cancer

These vitamins are present in a variety of foods and occur naturally in fruits and vegetables, which we should consume in plenty, especially when they are in season, whereas the intake of drugs, in comparison, is full of side-effects and they are no match for natural nutrients.

Let us analyse the components of antioxidants individually.

We stand an increasing risk from free radicals in our food. The main source is fats (such as cooking oils when they are heated to high temperatures). As fats are heated, their chemical structure breaks down to form peroxides. These peroxides further break down to form the dangerous hydroxyl radicals. This form of radicals is highly reactive and causes great damage to the cells and DNA.

(Poly-unsaturated fats such as sunflower and safflower oil are least stable at high temperatures. These become oxidized more quickly than mono-unsaturated fats such as olive oil).

Vitamin A

There are two main types of vitamin A, one found in animal products such as meat and milk which is called retinol and the other in fruits and vegetables called B-carotene. It is the B-carotene which acts as an antioxidant.

Vitamin A is needed for growth and for keeping the body tissues healthy. Its deficiency causes abnormality of skin and eyes and also retardation of healthy bone formation and good teeth condition. The deficiency may also lead to complete blindness if not treated in time. One of the most common causes of blindness in India is vitamin A deficiency. B-carotene is present in various coloured fruits and vegetables like spinach, coriander, amaranth, drumsticks, cabbage, carrots, mangoes, peaches, tomatoes etc. This carotene is converted into vitamin A in the body. B-carotene is not destroyed by cooking or by ultraviolet light; however only 30%-50% of B-carotene is absorbed.

Daily requirement for an adult is 600 mg of retinol or 2400 mg of B-carotene. Requirement for growing children, pregnant women and sick patients is higher. 1 mg B-carotene = 0.25 mg retinol.

However, prolonged intake of vitamin A in excess may cause toxic symptoms like headache, nausea, vomiting, drowsiness, anorexia, dry itchy skin, alopecia, cracking of lips etc.

In treating a patient, let your first thought be to strengthen his natural vitality.

— RHAZES

B-carotene works in two different ways. First it is converted into vitamin A by the body and the leftover B-carotene functions as an antioxidant. It is important not to confuse B-carotene with vitamin A, as these two are separate substances. There are two main types of vitamin A. One is found in foods derived from animals, such as meat and milk called retinol. The other is the carotenoid that is found in fruits and vegetables. There are around 600 of these, but the most important one is B-carotene. The body is able to convert B-carotene into vitamin A.

Vitamin A is needed for growth and for keeping the body tissues healthy. One of its most important roles is to reinforce the protective envelope or membrane that surrounds all our cells. It also protects the mucous membranes. It is fat-soluble. Fish liver oils are richest natural source of vitamin A.

B-carotene is a natural plant dye and was first discovered in carrots, hence the name given to the entire family was carotenoids. The carotenoids are a colourful range of pigments that provide the huge variety of paint box colours that we see in nature. B-carotene is a deep shade of red-orange and the main pigment in yellow and orange fruits and vegetables. Dark coloured vegetables of deep green also contain carotene but because of chlorophyll, the yellow or orange is masked. But sometimes the masking is not quite overbearing such as in the case of bitter gourd.

B-carotene is one of the most powerful antioxidants that prevent plants from burning up in the ultraviolet rays of the sun — nature's perfect antidote. Fruits and vegetables that contain B-carotene are melons, apricots, peaches, mangoes and carrots, parsley (raw), sweet potatoes, spinach, watercress (raw), spring onions, tomatoes, asparagus and broccoli.

Vitamin C (Ascorbic Acid)

Besides acting as an antioxidant, vitamin C possesses many

extraordinary properties. It helps in the growth and repair of body tissues, gums, blood vessels, bones and teeth. It is involved in the manual system and helps the body to fight off bacteria and viral infections. Deficiency of vitamin C is related to haemorrhage, slow healing of wounds, scurvy, gum bleeding, reduced formation of bones etc. Vitamin C is present in *amla*, the richest source of vitamin C, citrus fruits — lemon, *mosambi* (sweet lemon), orange, guava and green leafy vegetables like spinach.

Cooking and canning destroys vitamin C. Daily requirement for an adult is 40 mg/day. It is not stored in the body; excess amount is lost through urine.

Other men live to eat, while I eat to live.

— SOCRATES

Vitamin E

Vitamin E also acts as an antioxidant and is concentrated on the membranes and protects them from the action of peroxides. Vitamin E also protects vitamin A from oxidation and inhibits oxygen toxicity, thus being a scavenger of free radical oxygen. It strengthens the immune system by strengthening the white blood cells and helps in preventing heart diseases. Vitamin E is present in wheat germ, sprouts, whole grains, lettuce etc.

There are some trace elements which also work as antioxidants in our body e.g. Selenium, Molybdenum etc. However, we are not discussing them here.

Food items to be avoided

1. Milk (full cream) and milk products
2. Skimmed milk (*bina vasa ka doodh*) — beyond 200 ml

per day

3. Cheese and butter
4. Butter milk (*lassi*) beyond 200 ml of skimmed milk
5. All kinds of non-vegetarian items
6. Nuts and dry fruits
7. Sweets (*mithai*) which contain fat and oil
8. Oil (all types).

Food items moderately restricted

1. Brown and White Breads (Double Roti)
2. Rice (*Chawal*)
3. Vermicelli (*Sewain*)
4. Bajra
5. Jowar
6. Maize (*Makkai*)
7. Wheat *Chapati / Roti / Phulka*
8. Dry Peas (*Sukha Matar*)
9. Potato (*Alu*)
10. Sweet Potato (*Shakarkandi*),
11. Jaggery (*Gur*), Sugar (*Khandsari*)
12. Cane Sugar (*Chini*)
13. Ripe Banana (*Kela*)
14. Mango (*Aam*)
15. Cold Drinks
16. Thick Lentils (*Dal*)

Food items which can be consumed freely

Cereals
1. Puffed Rice (Murmura)
2. Rice Flakes (Chirwa, Poha)

Pulses
3. Bengal Gram Whole (Chana)
4. Bengal Gram Dal (Chana Dal)
5. Bengal Gram, roasted (Bhuna Chana)
6. Black Gram Dal (Urad Dal)
7. Cow Peas (Lobia)
8. Green Gram Whole (Moong Dal Sabut)
9. Green Gram Dal Split (Moong Dal Dhuli)
10. Horse Gram Whole (Kultha)
11. Lentil (Masoor /Tur)
12. Beans (Moth)
13. Green Peas (Matar)
14. Rajmah
15. Soyabean (Bhatmas)
16. Yellow Gram Dal (Arhal Dal)

Leafy Vegetables
17. Bathua Leaves (Bathua ka Saag)
18. Spinach (Palak)
19. Radish Leaves (Mooli ka Saag)
20. Cabbage (Patta Gobhi)
21. Amaranth (Cholai ka Saag)

22. Carrot Leaves *(Gajar ka Saag)*
23. Colocasia Leaves *(Arbi ka Saag)*
24. Drumsticks *(Saijan ki Phalli)*
25. Fenugreek Leaves *(Methi ka Saag)*
26. Lettuce *(Salad ka Patta)*
27. Mint *(Pudina)*
28. Mustard Leaves *(Sarson ka Saag)*

Roots and Tubers

29. Yam *(Jimikand)*
30. Carrots *(Gajar)*
31. Onions *(Pyaj)*
32. White Radish *(Safed Mooli)*
33. Garlic   *(Lehsun)*
34. Ginger *(Adrak)*

Other Vegetables

35. Beans *(Sem)*
36. Brinjal *(Baingan)*
37. Cucumber *(Khira)*
38. French Beans
39. Lotus Stem (Dry) *(Kamal Gatta)*
40. Pointed Gourd *(Parwal)*
41. Pumpkin *(Kaddu)*
42. Lady's Fingers *(Bhindi)*
43. Tinda
44. Ripe Tomatoes *(Tamatar)*
45. Bottle Gourd *(Ghia)*

46. Courgettes (*Torai*)

47. Capsicum (*Shimla Mirch*)

48. Kakri

49. Mushrooms (*Khumb*)

Fruits

50. Apple (*Seb*)

51. Guava (*Amrood*)

52. Lemon (*Nimbu*)

53. Sweet Lime (*Mosambi*)

54. Orange (*Santara*)

55. WaterMelon (*Tarbooj*)

56. Papaya Ripe (*Papita*)

57. Pineapple (*Ananas*)

58. Musk Melon (*Kharbooza*)

But if I am content with a little, enough is as good as a feast.

— Isaac Bickerstaffe

Nutritive value of Indian foods

(All the values are per 100 g of edible portion)

Foodstuff	Moisture (g)	Protein (g)	Fat (g)	CHO (g)	Fibre (g)	Energy (Kcal)
Cereals						
1. Bajra	12.4	11.6	5.0	67.5	1.2	361
2. Barley (*jau*)	12.5	11.5	1.3	69.6	3.9	336
3. Jowar	11.9	10.4	1.9	72.6	1.6	349
4. Maize (*makkai*)	14.9	11.1	3.6	66.2	2.7	342

Foodstuff	Moisture (g)	Protein (g)	Fat (g)	CHO (g)	Fibre (g)	Energy (Kcal)
5. Rice	13.7	6.8	0.5	78.2	0.2	345
6. Rice flakes	12.2	6.6	1.2	77.3	0.7	346
7. Rice (puffed)	14.7	7.5	0.1	73.6	0.3	325
8. Wheat (whole)	12.8	12.1	1.7	69.4	1.9	341
9. Wheat flour	12.2	12.1	1.7	69.4	1.9	341
10. Refined flour	13.3	11.0	0.9	73.9	0.3	348
11. Semolina (suji)	—	10.4	0.8	74.8	0.2	348
12. Vermicelli	11.7	8.7	0.4	78.3	0.2	352
13. Brown bread	39.0	8.8	1.4	49.0	1.2	244
14. White bread	39.0	7.8	0.7	51.9	0.2	245

Pulses

Foodstuff	Moisture (g)	Protein (g)	Fat (g)	CHO (g)	Fibre (g)	Energy (Kcal)
15. Bengal gram (whole)	9.8	17.1	5.3	60.9	3.9	360
16. Bengal gram dal	9.9	20.8	5.6	59.8	1.2	372
17. Roasted Bengal gram	10.7	22.5	5.2	58.1	1.0	369
18. Black gram dal	10.9	24.0	1.4	59.6	0.9	347
19. Cowpea (lobia)	13.4	24.1	1.0	54.5	3.8	323
20. Green gram (whole)	10.4	24.0	1.3	56.7	4.1	334
21. Green gram (dal)	10.1	24.5	1.2	59.9	0.8	348
22. Lentil	12.4	25.1	0.7	59.0	0.7	343
23. Moth beans	10.8	23.6	1.1	56.6	4.5	330
24. Peas (dry)	16.0	19.7	1.1	56.5	4.5	315
25. Rajmah	12.0	22.9	1.3	60.6	4.8	346
26. Red gram dal (masoor)	13.4	22.3	1.7	57.6	1.5	335
27. Soyabeans	8.1	43.2	19.5	20.9	3.7	432

Foodstuff	Moisture (g)	Protein (g)	Fat (g)	CHO (g)	Fibre (g)	Energy (Kcal)
Leafy Vegetables						
28. Beet greens	86.4	3.4	0.8	6.5	0.7	46
29. Brussel sprouts	85.5	4.7	0.5	7.1	1.2	52
30. Cabbage	91.9	1.8	0.1	4.6	1.0	27
31. Carrot leaves	76.6	5.1	0.5	13.1	1.9	77
32. Colocasia leaves	82.7	3.9	1.5	6.8	2.9	36
33. Coriander leaves	86.3	3.3	0.6	6.3	1.2	44
34. Curry leaves	63.8	6.1	1.0	18.7	6.4	108
35. Fenugreek leaves	86.1	4.4	0.9	6.0	1.1	49
36. Lettuce	93.4	2.1	0.3	2.5	0.5	21
37. Mint	84.9	4.8	0.6	5.8	2.0	48
38. Mustard leaves	89.8	4.0	0.6	3.2	0.8	34
39. Pigweed (*bathua*)	89.6	3.7	0.4	2.9	0.8	30
40. Radish leaves	90.8	3.8	0.4	2.4	1.0	28
41. Spinach	92.1	2.0	0.7	2.9	0.6	26
Roots and Tubers						
42. Beetroot	87.1	1.7	0.1	8.8	0.9	43
43. Carrot	86.0	0.9	0.2	10.6	1.2	48
44. Colocasia	73.1	3.0	0.1	21.1	1.0	97
45. Onion	84.3	1.8	0.1	12.6	0.6	59
46. Potato	74.7	1.6	0.1	22.6	0.4	97
47. Radish	94.4	0.7	0.1	3.4	0.8	17
48. Sweet potato	68.5	1.2	0.3	28.2	0.8	120
49. Tapioca	59.4	0.7	0.2	38.1	0.6	157
50. Turnip	91.6	0.5	0.2	6.2	0.9	29

Foodstuff	Moisture (g)	Protein (g)	Fat (g)	CHO (g)	Fibre (g)	Energy (Kcal)
Other Vegetables						
51. Bitter gourd	92.4	1.6	0.2	4.2	0.8	25
52. Bottle gourd (*lauki*)	96.1	0.2	0.1	2.5	0.6	12
53. Brinjal	92.7	1.4	0.3	4.0	1.3	24
54. Broad beans	85.4	4.5	0.1	7.2	2.0	48
55. Capsicum	92.4	1.3	0.3	4.3	1.0	24
56. Cauliflower	90.8	2.6	0.4	4.0	1.2	30
57. Cucumber	96.3	0.4	0.1	2.5	0.4	13
58. Drumsticks	86.9	2.5	0.1	3.7	4.8	26
59. French beans	91.4	1.7	0.1	4.5	1.8	26
60. Jackfruit tender (*kathal*)	84.0	2.6	0.3	9.4	2.8	51
61. Lady's fingers	89.6	1.9	0.2	6.4	1.2	35
62. Lotus stem (dry)	9.5	4.1	1.3	51.4	25.0	234
63. Mango (green)	87.5	0.7	0.1	10.1	1.2	44
64. Onion stalks	87.6	0.1	0.2	8.9	1.6	41
65. Plantain (green)	83.2	1.4	0.2	14.0	0.7	64
66. Pointed gourd (*parwal*)	92.0	2.0	0.3	2.2	3.0	20
67. Pumpkin (*kaddu*)	92.6	1.4	0.1	4.6	0.7	25
68. Ridge gourd (*kali tori*)	95.2	0.5	0.1	3.4	0.5	17
69. Tinda	93.5	1.4	0.2	3.4	1.0	21
70. Tomato (green)	93.1	1.9	0.1	3.6	0.7	23
71. Water chestnuts	70.0	4.7	0.3	23.3	0.6	115
Nuts and Oilseeds						
72. Almonds	5.2	20.8	58.9	10.5	1.7	655
73. Arecanut (*supari*)	31.3	4.9	4.4	47.2	11.2	249
74. Cashewnuts	5.9	21.2	46.9	22.3	1.3	596

Foodstuff	Moisture (g)	Protein (g)	Fat (g)	CHO (g)	Fibre (g)	Energy (Kcal)
75. Coconut (dry)	4.3	6.8	62.3	18.4	66.6	662
76. Coconut (fresh)	36.3	4.5	41.6	13.0	3.6	444
77. Coconut (tender)	90.8	0.9	1.4	6.3	-	41
78. Coconut milk	42.8	3.4	41.0	11.9	-	430
79. Coconut water	93.8	1.4	0.1	4.4	-	24
80. Gingelly seeds (til)	5.3	18.3	43.3	25.0	2.9	563
81. Groundnuts	3.0	25.3	40.1	26.1	3.1	567
82. Groundnuts (roasted)	1.7	26.2	39.8	26.7	3.1	570
83. Pine nuts (chilgoza)	4.0	13.9	49.3	29.0	1.0	615
84. Mustard seeds	8.5	20.0	39.7	23.8	1.8	541
85. Pistachio nuts	5.6	19.8	53.5	16.2	2.1	626
86. Sapid nuts (chironji)	3.0	19.0	59.1	12.1	3.8	656
87. Walnuts	4.5	15.6	64.5	11.0	2.6	687

Spices

Foodstuff	Moisture (g)	Protein (g)	Fat (g)	CHO (g)	Fibre (g)	Energy (Kcal)
88. Asafoetida (hing)	16.0	4.0	1.1	67.8	4.1	297
89. Cardamoms	20.0	10.2	2.2	42.1	20.1	229
90. Chillies (red, dry)	10.0	15.9	6.2	31.6	30.2	246
91. Chillies (green)	85.7	2.9	0.6	3.0	6.8	29
92. Cloves	25.2	5.2	8.9	46.0	9.5	286
93. Coriander	11.2	14.1	16.1	21.6	32.6	288
94. Cumin seeds	11.9	18.7	15.0	36.6	12.0	356
95. Fenugreek seeds	13.7	26.2	5.8	44.1	7.2	333
96. Garlic	62.0	6.3	0.1	29.8	0.8	145
97. Ginger	80.9	2.3	0.9	12.3	2.4	67
98. Mango powder (amchoor)	6.8	2.8	7.8	64.0	13.7	337

Foodstuff	Moisture (g)	Protein (g)	Fat (g)	CHO (g)	Fibre (g)	Energy (Kcal)
99. Black pepper (*kali mirch*)	18.2	11.5	6.8	49.2	14.9	304
100. Poppy seeds (*khus khus*)	4.3	21.7	19.3	36.8	8.0	408
101. Tamarind pulp	20.9	3.1	0.1	67.4	5.6	283
102. Turmeric	13.31	6.3	5.1	69.4	2.6	349

Fruits

Foodstuff	Moisture (g)	Protein (g)	Fat (g)	CHO (g)	Fibre (g)	Energy (Kcal)
103. Amla	81.8	0.5	0.1	13.7	3.4	58
104. Apple	84.6	0.2	0.5	13.4	1.0	59
105. Apricot, (fresh)	85.3	1.0	0.3	11.6	1.1	53
106. Apricot (dry)	19.4	1.6	0.7	73.4	2.1	306
107. Ball fruit	61.5	1.8	0.3	31.8	2.9	137
108. Cape gooseberry (*rasbhari*)	82.9	1.8	0.2	11.1	3.2	53
109. Cherries	83.4	1.1	0.5	13.8	0.4	64
110. Currants (block) (*munakka*)	18.4	2.7	0.5	75.2	1.0	316
111. Custard apple (*sharifa*)	70.5	1.6	0.4	23.5	3.1	104
112. Dates (fresh)	59.2	1.2	0.4	33.8	3.7	144
113. Figs (*anjeer*)	88.1	1.3	0.2	7.6	2.2	37
114. Grapes	79.2	0.5	0.3	16.5	2.9	751
115. Guava	81.7	0.9	0.3	11.2	5.2	51
116. Jackfruit (*kathal*)	76.2	1.9	0.1	19.8	1.1	88
117. Jamun	83.7	0.7	0.3	14.0	0.9	62
118. Lemon	85.0	1.0	0.9	11.1	1.7	57
119. Lichi	84.1	1.1	0.2	13.6	0.5	61

Foodstuff	Moisture (g)	Protein (g)	Fat (g)	CHO (g)	Fibre (g)	Energy (Kcal)
120. Malta	90.3	0.7	0.2	7.8	0.6	36
121. Mango	81.0	0.6	0.4	16.9	0.7	74
122. Musk melon	95.2	0.3	0.2	3.5	0.4	17
123. Orange	87.6	0.7	0.2	10.9	0.3	48
124. Papaya	90.8	0.6	0.1	7.2	0.8	32
125. Peaches (aarhoo)	86.0	1.2	0.3	10.5	1.2	50
126. Pears (nashpati)	86.0	0.6	0.2	11.9	1.0	52
127. Phalsa	80.8	1.3	0.9	14.7	1.2	72
128. Pineapple	87.8	(−)	0.1	10.8	0.5	46
129. Plum (Alu bokhara)	86.9	0.7	0.5	11.1	0.4	52
130. Pomegranate (Anaar)	78.0	1.6	0.1	14.5	5.1	65
131. Raisins (Kishmish)	20.2	1.8	0.3	74.6	1.1	3048
132. Sapota (chiku)	73.7	0.7	1.1	21.4	2.6	98
133. Strawberry	87.8	0.7	0.2	9.8	1.1	44
134. Sweet Lemon (mosambi)	88.4	0.8	0.3	9.3	0.5	43
135. Tomato	94.0	0.9	0.2	3.6	0.8	20
136. Water-melon	95.8	0.2	0.2	3.3	0.2	16
137. Wood apple (bael)	70.1	1.2	0.3	21.2	0.4	116
138. Zizyphus (ber)	81.6	0.8	0.3	17.0	-	74

Milk and Milk Products

Foodstuff	Moisture (g)	Protein (g)	Fat (g)	CHO (g)	Fibre (g)	Energy (Kcal)
139. Milk (Buffalo's)	81.0	4.3	6.5	5.0	-	117
140. Milk (Cow's)	87.5	3.2	4.1	4.4	-	67
141. Milk (Goat's)	86.8	3.3	4.5	4.6	-	72
142. Curd (Cow's milk)	89.1	3.1	4.0	3.0	-	60
143. Butter milk	97.5	0.8	1.1	0.5	-	15
144. Sk. milk (Liquid)	92.1	2.5	0.1	4.6	-	29

Foodstuff	Moisture (g)	Protein (g)	Fat (g)	CHO (g)	Fibre (g)	Energy (Kcal)
145. *Chhenna*, (Cow's milk)	57.1	18.3	20.8	1.2	-	265
146. *Chhenna*, (Buffalo's milk)	54.1	13.4	23.0	7.9	-	292
147. *Khoya* (Buffalo's milk)	30.6	14.6	31.2	20.5	-	421
148. *Khoya* (Cow's milk)	25.2	20.0	25.9	24.9	-	413
149. Skimmed milk powder (Cow's milk)	4.1	38.0	0.1	51.0	-	357
150. Whole milk powder (Cow's milk)	3.5	25.8	26.7	38.0	-	497

Fats and Oils

Foodstuff	Moisture (g)	Protein (g)	Fat (g)	CHO (g)	Fibre (g)	Energy (Kcal)
151. Butter	19.0	-	-	81.0	-	729
152. *Ghee*/Oils	-	-	100.0	-	-	900

Sugars

Foodstuff	Moisture (g)	Protein (g)	Fat (g)	CHO (g)	Fibre (g)	Energy (Kcal)
153. Sugar	0.4	0.1	-	99.4	-	398
154. Honey	20.6	0.3	-	79.5	-	319
155. Jaggery	3.9	0.4	0.1	95.0	-	383
156. Sago	12.2	0.2	0.2	87.1	-	3 5 1

Source: **Nutritive Value of Indian Foods, NIN, Indian Council of Medical Research**

The oil controversy

Let me mention in this chapter details about oils and clear some of the misconceptions for you.

Going by the way the oil companies advertise it appears that some oils should be really good for the blockages. The scientific name of oil is triglycerides. If you take any standard oil it is almost 100% fat i.e. triglycerides. To underplay this overwhelming concentration of fats in most oils, the manufacturers use different ways to impress upon consumers about the different fatty acids which make triglycerides.

Let me explain: tri of triglycerides means three; glyceride comes from glycerol. Triglycerides is composed of one molecule (small unit) of glycerol and 3 fatty chains (called fatty acids). These fatty acids present in the triglycerides can be of three kinds — poly-unsaturated, mono-unsaturated and saturated fatty acids. If one hydrogen is absent it is called mono-unsaturated and if more than one hydrogen is absent it is poly-unsaturated. The difference between these three, in terms of composition or side-effects is almost the same. For example, if saturated fatty acids is 92% harmful, mono will be 90% and poly will be 88%. This is not clear to the public and the oil companies take advantage of it.

Take for example, one oil which has 70% poly-unsaturated, 25% mono-unsaturated and 5% saturated, will have in all 100% triglycerides content. To advertise the company writes "95% saturated FAT FREE", the last two in bold and so is 95%. For people who do not understand saturated or mono-unsaturated — this advertisement appears as if the oil has only 5% fat and they consume that particular oil in large quantities without understanding that it has 100% fat, out of which 95% are mono and poly type fat. Legally the oil companies cannot be punished. Heart patients fall into the trap more easily as these companies also write "CHOLESTEROL" Free. This is going on since cardiologists have accepted these and oil companies sponsor the doctor's meets.

You would probably ask, "Doctor, what about your recommended oil?" I have none. I offer water for cooking food. That is what is zero oil. You may also ask, what about the body's oil requirement. National Institute of Nutrition (NIN) — the prime body of government for food recommends that a minimum of

10% of calories required in our body should come from fat. If we take this figure at 1600 calories per day then 160 calories should come from fat. This will make about 18 to 20 gms per day of minimal fat requirement. SAAOL recommends only this quantity to heart patients who want to reverse there ailments, but in a normal person's diet, this fat comes automatically from hidden fats in cereals and pulses. So, we do not require any further addition of raw oil to our diet.

When you have faults, do not fear to abandon them.

— CONFUCIUS

Oils and their composition

	Name	Saturated	Mono-unsaturated	Poly-unsaturated
1.	Coconut oil	86	6	2
2.	Ghee (Buffalo)	74	19	3
3.	Ghee (Cow)	71	25	2
4.	Vanaspati	76	19	3.5
5.	Olive oil	14	72	2
6.	Palm oil	48	38	10
7.	Groundnut oil	19	47	30
8.	Sesame oil	15	39	41
9.	Corn oil	13	25	58
10.	Sunflower oil	11	34	50
11.	Safflower oil	9	12	74
12.	Rapeseed oil	4	11	82
13.	Mustard oil	4	11	82
14.	Soyabean oil	15	23	59

Source : Bulletin, NIN, Hyderabad, India.
The percentages do not add up to 100% as an average value is taken.

Invisible fat content of food items

(per 100 gm)

Name	Invisible Fat Content (g)
1. Bajra	5
2. Maize	3.6
3. Rice	0.5 - 1
4. Wheat	1.5
5. Bengal gram	5.3
6. Green peas	0.1
7. Rajmah	1.3
8. Green leaves	0.1 - 0.5
9. Carrot	0.2
10. Onion	0.1
11. Potato	0.1
12. Radish	0.1
13. Brinjal	0.3
14. Cauliflower	0.4
15. Green mango	0.1
16. Tomato	0.1
17. Almonds	58.9
18. Cashewnuts	46.9
19. Coconut water	0.1
20. Coconut (fresh)	41.6
21. Groundnuts	40.1
22. Green chillies	0.6
23. Garlic	0.1
24. Apple	0.5
25. Banana	0.3
26. Dates	0.4
27. Fish	0.1 - 0.2
28. Beef	10.3

Name	Invisible Fat Content (g)
29. Egg	13.3
30. Mutton	29.0
31. Buffalo's Milk	6.5
32. Cow's Milk	4.1
33. Curd	4.0
34. Butter-milk	1.1
35. Chhenna	20.0 - 25.0
35. Khoa	31
36. Butter	81
37. All oils	100
38. Sugar	0
39. Honey	0

Tips

❑ Garlic is found to lower blood pressure, prevent coronary thrombosis, heart attacks and strokes, diabetes, yeast infections, allergies and stress. It has also been found to inhibit the growth of cancerous tumours.

❑ Garlic is a classic example of a combination of food and folk medicine. It boosts immune response and increases resistance against various diseases. It also has antibacterial, antifungal and antithrombic effects.

❑ For suppressing the strong odour of garlic, parsley can be chewed along with it.

❑ Honey is a good substitute for sugar. It is sweeter than sugar and is absorbed more quickly. Unlike sugar it contains vitamin B, some minerals and enzymes in addition.

❑ To prepare tofu: Soak dried soyabeans in water till soft, then crush and boil. Strain and separate the pulp and soyamilk. To this milk add lemon or citric or tartaric acid. The milk curdles into curd and whey. Put the curd into a mould for setting. Within 2-3 hours, tofu is ready.

❑ Lemon is an excellent source of vitamin C and also contains some amount of calcium, phosphorus, potassium and carotene. It is also found to be an antiseptic. It can be easily used as a low calorie salad dressing.

❑ Cardamom is mainly used as a cooking spice or for flavouring drinks. It is known as a carminative, relieving flatulence, stimulation for stomach and aiding digestion.

❑ Cut vegetables into small pieces as the flavour will be extracted easily in 20 minutes. If you cut them larger you will need to cook them longer to extract its flavour.

❑ It is not difficult to make delicious food without adding fat. Make judicious use of spices and herbs, which can help in making dishes tasty and varied. Their intense flavour can compensate for lack of fat.

❑ Cut down on salt.

❑ Add salt at table rather than while cooking, you will need less for taste and thus less consumption.

❑ Use other flavourings in food like garlic, lemon juice, vinegar, tomato, herbs and spices.

❑ Avoid food with high salt content, such as pickles.

❑ Like all tastes, salt is also an acquired taste.

❑ Fresh herbs should be added at the last minute for maximum flavour and save a sprig or two for garnishing.

❑ Dried herbs need to be stewed for few minutes before they change their character.

- Read food labels for calorie and fat contents and avoid products with added sugar.

- Avoid tasting dishes too often. 3-4 spoonfuls of a sauce or gravy can contain a surprising number of calories. If you want taste, use a teaspoon.

- Never add acidic foods like tomatoes, lemon juice to beans until the beans are soft. The acid can keep the beans from softening.

- Mushrooms are fungi rich in potassium, phosphorus, copper and iron. They are also a good source of vitamin B_1 and B_2. They are known to be beneficial in reducing blood fat levels, have antibiotic properties, antitumour activity and boost immune system against diseases producing micro-organisms.

- Mustard is a popular culinary herb that stimulates the appetite and helps digestion.

- Onion, alongwith its culinary property, helps to prevent blood clot and heart attacks. It has also shown to lower high blood pressure and cholesterol levels.

- Papaya is known for its ability to aid digestion. It contains enzymes that help to digest proteins. Papaya is a rich source of beta-carotene, vitamin B and vitamin C.

- Potato is a good source of vegetable protein, potassium, vitamin C, iron, phosphorus and enzymes. It relieves water retention and can sometimes be used to reduce hypertension and promote intestinal flora.

- Pumpkin is a good source of beta-carotene, calcium, iron and some vitamin B. It helps to regulate blood sugar levels and is thus beneficial to hypoglycemics.

- Spinach is an excellent source of iron, calcium, chlorophyll, beta-carotene, vitamin C, riboflavin, sodium and potassium.

It is also a diuretic and laxative.

- Sprouts are rich in chlorophyll, vitamin A, C, D, E, K and B complexes and in minerals such as calcium, phosphorus, potassium, magnesium and iron.

- Sprout are diuretics, appetizers and help detoxify the body.

- Turmeric is not used as seasoning but also as a food preservative and colouring agent. It also has unique antioxidant and anti-inflamatory properties. It retards age related diseases by preventing free radical damage, inhibits growth of cancer cells, protects liver from cholesterol levels, alleviates joint swellings, reduces menstrual pain and has a beneficial effect in the treatment of AIDS.

- As with any other nutrient the body requires water in balanced amounts. Too much water particularly after meals will dilute digestive juices, weaken digestion and cause a sensation of coldness. On the other hand, insufficient water intake will promote constipation, accumulation of toxins, kidney damage, fatigue, apathy and dryness.

- Grains and legumes when cooked contain about 80% water, many fruits and vegetables contain over 90% water, while, the content of soups and juices is almost 100% water.

- Nutritional benefit of curd is to reinforce the intestines with additional friendly bacteria promoting the growth of intestines flora. It is a good source of quality proteins, vitamins and is an excellent source of easily absorbed calcium. It is easily digestible.

- Start your meals with a bowl of low-fat, high-protein soup. It will satiate your appetite, and you'll probably eat less amount of the fattening foods that may follow. But beware of cream-based soups — they're more fatty than most.

- Eat your meals slowly. Gulping your food is bad for digestion.

If you put down your eating utensils (spoon fork) between each bite, you will chew your food more thoroughly and enjoy it more.

Typical Diet Contains

40-50 % fats (mostly saturated)

25-35 % carbohydrates

25 % proteins

400-500 mg cholesterol per day.

The Reversal Diet Contains

10 % fats (invisible form)

70-75 % carbohydrates

15-20 % proteins

10 mg cholesterol per day

Cholesterol: the main culprit

Cholesterol Content of Food

Food	Quantity (g)	Household Measures	Cholesterol Content (mg)
Meat and its Products			
Yellow of eggs	100 g	2	420
Chicken (broiler)	100 g	1 portion	60
Mutton (goat) (Medium fat/lean)	100 g	3-4 pieces	65
Liver	100 g	4-6 pieces	300
Kidney	100 g	1 piece	150
Brain	100 g	7 tbsp	250
Pork	100 g	1 slice	70

Food	Quantity (g)	Household Measures	Cholesterol Content (mg)
Oysters	100 g	1 portion	230-470
Shrimps	100 g	1 portion	150
Crab	100 g	1 portion	145
Pork ribs	100 g	2	105
Lamb	100 g	1 portion	70

Milk and Milk Products

Whole milk	100 ml	1 small cup	11
Skimmed milk	100 ml	1 small cup	2.4
Cream	100 ml	1 small cup	100
Butter	100 g	1 small cup	240
Cheese	100 g	4 slices	16
Plain ice cream	100 g	1 small cup	375
Animal fat	100 g	1 small cup	90

Some heart friendly recipes

Sprouted Dal Salad

Ingredients:

50 gm any sprouted dal

1 small onion (finely chopped)

1 small tomato (chopped)

Fresh coriander leaves (finely chopped)

Green chillies (chopped)

$1/_4$ tsp salt

$^1/_4$ tsp black salt

$^1/_2$ tsp roasted cumin seeds

$^1/_2$ tsp amchoor (dry mango powder)

$^1/_4$ tsp red chilli powder

Juice of 1 lemon

1. Soften the sprouted dal in very little water (for 2-3 minutes).
2. To this dal, add all the ingredients.
3. While serving sprinkle the coriander leaves.

Sweet Lime and Cucumber Salad

1 tsp gelatin

200 ml sweet lime juice

$^1/_2$ cucumber (grated)

Salt and black pepper according to taste

1. Add the gelatin to $^1/_4$ cup of sweet lime juice and warm it a little.
2. When cool, add the remaining juice and refrigerate it.
3. Take it out after 15-20 minutes or when set. Add it to the grated cucumber.
4. Put this mixture in the empty peels of the sweet lime.
5. Again refrigerate it.

Kabuli and Kala Chana Salad

25 gm Kabuli and kala chana (soaked overnight)

1 small capsicum (chopped)

1 small onion

1 small tomato

1 tsp finely grated ginger

Finely chopped coriander and green chillies

Salt to taste

$^1/_4$ tsp black salt

$^1/_4$ tsp black pepper

$^1/_2$ tsp sugar

A pinch of mustard powder

$^1/_2$ tsp chaat masala

$^1/_2$ tsp cumin seed powder (roasted)

1 tsp lemon juice

1. Boil the soaked chanas.
2. Add all the ingredients to the boiled chanas.
3. Serve garnished with chopped coriander leaves and green chillies.

Stuffed Pear Salad

6 large pears

150 gm black grapes

1 cup curd

1 tsp sugar

Salt and black pepper to taste

1. Tie the curd in a thin muslin cloth to drain away the extra water (for at least 3 hrs).

2. Peel the pears and cut them into 2 halves. Scoop out the inner part (pears look like cups when cut).

3. Cut the grapes and take out the pips, if any. Mix with pear pulp.

4. To the curd add sugar and salt.

5. Put this mixture of grapes and curd into each pear cup.

6. Serve chilled.

Minestrone Soup

2 onions medium sized

1 carrot

1 potato

6 to 7 French beans

2 medium sized tomatoes

$^1/_2$ cup finely chopped cabbage

1 bay leaf tejpatta

$^1/_2$ cup boiled noodles

3 tsp boiled kidney beans (rajmah)

Salt and black pepper to taste

1. Dice the tomatoes, finely chop the cabbage, cut onion rings and cut the rest of the vegetables into slender pieces.

2. Dry roast the onions, French beans, carrots for at least 3 minutes.

3. Boil 6 cups of water. Add the bay leaf to it.

4. Now add the potato, cabbage and tomatoes.

> I feel a recipe is only a theme, which an intelligent cook can play each time with a variation.
>
> — MADAME BENOIT

5. Boil for another 10-15 minutes.

6. To this add the noodles, boiled rajmah, salt and black pepper.

7. Serve hot.

Cabbage Soup

For the stock

25 gm cabbage
225 gm bottle gourd (lauki)
2 medium onions
2 potatoes
Salt and black pepper to taste

For the decoration
1 finely chopped onion
1 carrot finely sliced
$^1/_2$ cup finely chopped cabbage

Stock

1. Cut all the vegetables into big cubes. Add 7 cups of water and pressure-cook it.

2. When cooked keep aside.

Preparation

3. In a pan add all the finely chopped vegetables with stock and cook for at least 20 minutes.

4. Add salt and black pepper to taste.

5. Serve hot.

Beetroot Soup

2 medium sized beetroots

> A man is satisfied not by the quality of food but by the absense of greed.
> — GURDJIEFF

1 tsp maize flour

1 tsp finely chopped onion

1 tsp lemon juice

1 tsp vinegar

Salt and black pepper to taste.

1. Skin, grate and boil the beetroots and keep aside.
2. Dry roast the maize flour till golden brown. Keep aside.
3. Sauté the onion till light brown. To this add water (a little extra than the cups of soup you want), beetroot and salt. Cook for 10-15 minutes.
4. Transfer this to a liquidizer. Blend properly and strain.
5. Reboil the mixture.
6. Remove from heat. Add lemon juice, vinegar and black pepper to the soup.
7. Serve hot.

Stuffed Rotis

Carrots/ radish/ potato/ beans/ cabbage/ cauliflower/ fenugreek/ spinach/ dal — (anyone)

Wheat flour

Gram flour (besan)

Garam masala

Salt

Red chilli powder

1. Whatever vegetable is to be used for the stuffing has to be boiled and mashed.
2. Mix the wheat and gram flours together. Now add the

masalas and stuffing to this.

3. Knead the flour and roll out *rotis* and roast them on the *tava* or griddle.

4. Serve hot with tomato or green chutney.

Chana Dal Bhel

100 gm chana dal

1 small piece ginger

1-2 gm finely chopped green chillies

$^1/_2$ small onion finely chopped

2 garlic cloves finely chopped

$^1/_2$ tsp mustard seeds powder

$^3/_4$ tsp sour curd

$^1/_2$-1 tsp lemon juice

$^1/_2$-1 tsp sugar (ground)

a pinch of asafoetida

$^1/_4$ tsp black pepper

6-7 curry leaves

salt to taste

$^1/_4$ tsp soda bicarb

A pinch of turmeric

finely chopped coriander leaves

1. Soak the chana dal overnight. Drain the water in the morning.

2. Take $^1/_2$ the dal. Add to it

> The biggest seller is cookbooks and the second is diet books — how not to eat what you've just learned how to cook.
>
> — ANDY ROONEY

the ginger, green chillies, curd and grind it coarsely.

3. Add to this mixture the remaining whole dal along with salt and turmeric powder. Keep this mixture covered for 6 hours.

4. Add soda bicarb, lemon juice and sugar to the mixture.

5. Put this mixture on an idli stand and steam-cook it.

6. When cooked, cool and crumble it.

7. Take 1 teaspoonful add a little asafoetida and mustard powder to it and heat it. Add this to the crumbled mixture.

8. In a pan, sauté garlic and onion till golden brown. To this add the curry leaves and mix into the crumbled mixture.

9. Before serving garnish with coriander leaves.

Dal

Any dal

1 small chopped onion

1 small chopped tomato

1 tsp ginger-garlic paste

$1/_2$ tsp turmeric

$1/_2$ tsp red chilli powder

$1/_2$ tsp garam masala

Salt to taste

1. Boil the dal with salt and turmeric in a cooker.

2. In a *karahi* add onion. Roast till golden brown, to this add the ginger-garlic paste, tomato, salt, chili powder and garam masala.

3. When the gravy is ready add it to the dal.

4. Let the dal come to a boil again.

5. Serve sprinkled with fresh coriander leaves.

Dal Dhokli

50 gm any washed dal

25 gm spinach

$\frac{1}{4}$ tsp turmeric powder

1 clove garlic

$\frac{1}{2}$ tsp red chilli powder

$\frac{1}{2}$ tsp cumin seeds

$\frac{1}{2}$ tsp garam masala powder

A pinch asafoetida

Salt to taste

2 cups water

Juice of 1 lemon

1 tsp sugar

1 cup tamarind chutney or tamarind water

4 gm paneer or any other vegetable for stuffing

1 cup wheat flour

1. Wash the dal. Add to it turmeric powder, salt and spinach and cook it for 5 minutes in the cooker.

2. To a pan add cumin seeds, turmeric and red chilli powders, salt and garam masala powder and roast them, then add the tamarind chutney or water and cook.

3. Knead a stiff dough with wheat flour to which a little red chilli powder is added.

4. Now roll out 2 to 3 thin rotis. Cut these rotis into 4 parts each. Stuff the paneer/vegetable as desired and keep aside.

5. Add the prepared rotis (dhoklis) to boiling masala water and cook for 20 minutes.

6. When cooked add them to the dal.

Kofta Curry

100 gm bottle gourd (lauki)

25 gm gram flour (besan)

Salt to taste

$^1/_2$ tsp red chilli powder

$^1/_2$ tsp garam masala

$^1/_2$ tsp mango powder (amchoor)

$^1/_2$ tsp turmeric powder

1. Grate the bottle gourd. Put it in a little water and boil it properly.

2. Dry roast the *besan*.

3. Drain excessive water from the bottle gourd. Add *besan*, salt, red chilli powder, garam masala and mix well. Make small balls out of the mixture.

4. Boil some water in a pan. Cover it with a sieve. Keep the balls (*koftas*) on it. Cover it properly. Cook till done.

5. Make onion-tomato gravy and add it to the steamed balls (*koftas*) and cook.

6. Serve hot sprinkled with fresh coriander leaves.

Saag

Spinach / mustard / bathua

Onion (finely chopped)

Tomato (chopped)

Onion-garlic paste

gram flour (besan)

Salt to taste

Red chilli powder

1. Boil the vegetables and mash.

2. In a *karahi* roast the chopped onion till golden brown and add tomato to it. Cook till the tomato is tender.

3. To this add the boiled and mashed vegetable.

4. Now on the *tava* dry-roast the *besan*.

5. When the vegetable is almost done add *besan* and cook for some more time.

6. Serve hot.

Dry vegetables with gram flour

1 cup gram flour

1 finely chopped medium size onion

1 medium size potato, cut into small pieces

2 tomatoes, cut into small pieces

3 to 4 pieces cauliflower florets

Finely chopped coriander leaves

2 green chillies

2 dry whole red chillies

1 tsp mustard seeds

1 sprig curry leaves

salt to taste

$1/_4$ tsp red chilli powder

1. Roast the gram flour till golden brown on slow flame and keep aside.

2. Roast the mustard seeds, curry leaves and whole red chillies and keep aside.

3. Take a pan with 1 cup of water to which a little salt is added. Add the chopped onion, potato and cauliflower to it and cook till soft.

4. When the vegetables are soft add the gram flour, chopped green chillies and red chilli powder. Cook on a low flame till the water dries.

5. Add the tomatoes and cook for another 3 to 4 minutes.

6. Serve hot decorated with tomatoes, green chillies and corriander leaves.

Section 10

Role of Yoga in Reversal

Contents

Yoga: the best science possible

Yoga and relaxation have been successfully used for the amelioration of high blood pressure and coronary heart disease over the past few decades. Recent research has proved that this form of treatment not only reduces high blood pressure but also reduces the serum cholesterol levels, serum triglyceride levels, serum free fatty acid, blood glucose, body weight and coronary artery disease. No form of medicine is as effective in the treatment of coronary heart disease as yoga. Moreover, this form of therapy has no side effects unlike medical drugs. Yogic practice also improves physical fitness and helps to improve an individual's efficiency. In SAAOL, we are using a particular lifestyle enhancement intervention based on *Preksha* yoga.

The most important plus point of yoga is that it takes the body and mind as a single unit. In medical science the body is divided into so many divisions and every division has its specialists. No doubt, this compartmentalisation of the body has its own advantages but when you treat the heart, you should not forget about the stomach. When you give a chemical for treating the infection in the lungs, it may have some side-effects on the kidney or liver. This has now created problems for medical science. They have forgotten to take the body as a single unit, with all the organs working in co-ordination. Our blood flow goes to every organ of the body every minute, so before putting a chemical in this bloodstream you must know its effects on all the organs wherever the blood reaches.

On the other hand, yoga is a positive therapy. When it works on the joints, it has a positive effect on the muscles and the mind. When it treats the heart, it also solves the stomach problem. When it lowers cholesterol, it also helps in increasing flexibility. When it is used to treat asthma, it also works on cervical spondylosis. It has good effects on all the other organs of the body.

Thus, when we use yoga as a therapy, it has a tremendous advantage over medical science, now considered as the science of the chemicals and knives.

Medical science has failed to understand yoga

Medical science has one great positive factor. It has a lot of information about the human body, its functions and it is based on reasoning and proofs. It has progressed because it makes an analysis of everything on the basis of available information and creates a vast infrastructure. It tries to put everything in black and white. The spread has been so vast and organised that, in spite of its shortcomings, it has become the number one cover for almost 99% percent of the world population.

This has not been done by the yoga experts. Thus this great science has not been able to spread to the masses in an organised way. Most of the medical doctors look down upon yoga as an unscientific way to deal with the human body because there was no one to study yoga deeply and explain its features to the medical doctors in the language they understood. Research studies and patients' data are what the medical science wants. It needs to know the improvements in terms of objective figures, which can be quantified or measured and then reproduced over and over again.

The problem is that yoga experts have not tried to learn medical science and medical doctors have not tried to go deep into the science of yoga. There has been no communication. Both speak in their own way and no understanding has developed between them.

But newly detected faults of medical science have compelled us to look into yoga. As it is a science of the body, yoga has the answers to stress management, to diseases which are due to lack of communication between the body and the mind. The use of chemicals and knives on the brain has tremendous side-effects. It would almost threaten the body's existence, the fact that medical science understood. They did not have the technology to work on the mind. They found that yoga seems to have an answer. Yoga can treat the mind or the brain — which is the site of all stresses and origin of the life-style related diseases. So they now want to adopt yoga as a part of medical science, of course by default. They are hardly left with any option.

Medical science needs all the proofs recorded and quantified, as per the rules to adopt the science of yoga, . It needs to record the parameter called stress which till now they could not do with the existing technology. Their technology fell short. They did not have people who would leave their lucrative practice of medicine or surgery and read all the literature on yoga, mostly in Sanskrit and local languages. There was no one who could explain to them all about yoga in totality. The very first thing they needed was a definition, which was also not available. The process went on slowly.

In the meantime, during this delay, the chemical manufacturers (drug companies) and the surgical manufacturers almost took over medical science. The body's physiology and normal functioning was deliberately overpowered. Something unphysiological and unnatural took over medical science. The surgery and chemical treatment was overdone. The future of this ongoing chemical treatment is sealed because its basis is completely wrong, unethical, biased and will boomerang.

This wrong diversification of medical science is also one of the reasons why yogic science could not be a part of modern medical science. Both were completely opposed to each other.

There was a clash all the time. One wanted to cut open the body, use chemicals whereas the other one wanted to use the body's normal existing superb mechanism to cure itself. Both wanted to work on the same diseases, the common diseases. The profitability of the former, because of the organisation and infrastructure, seems to be edging till now against the latter. But the truth lies with the second, which is still slow in the race, and has failed to convince medical science. They could not convince because the instruments of medical science were not advanced enough to understand the benefits of yoga.

It should be the function of medicine to have people die young as late as possible.
— ERNST L WYNDER, MD

What is yoga?

Definition

Yoga is the philosophical doctrine developed in India about 500 BC. It is based on moral principles, meditational techniques and a special type of physical training called hatha yoga which involves control of posture and respiration. It is said to bring about the right interaction, combination, co-ordination of the mind and body.

Other Definitions

❑ Union between prana (vital force) and maha shakti (universal energy)

❑ Stopping of fluctuations or disturbances of the conscious mind (Chitta).

❑ Achievement of inner equilibrium (Samatvam) harmony.

❑ Yoga is the skill of work (कर्मसु कौशलम्).

Faults of Yoga: Erratic Claims

Yogic science has not done much of an analysis about how its system works, on which organ does it work and what hormones it can secrete and so on. Most of the therapy was available, they have used it without a trained person or someone who has studied it thoroughly. Most of the yoga teachers are there by default. They could not become medical doctors or businessmen or may be engineers — so they have ventured into yoga. They neither have any understanding of the body nor a complete knowledge about their great science. Many yoga teachers or yoga doctors teach yoga as recreation or as a hobby, whenever they are free.

Eight steps of yoga

Yoga is one of the oldest sciences, as old as 5000 years. It has been described inthe earliest epics like the Vedas and Agams. Rishi Patanjali, father of yoga (300 BC) is the most widely known yoga guru. According to Patanjali there are 8 steps of yoga, viz. yam (यम्) niyama (नियम) asana (आसन), pranayama (प्राणायाम), pratyahar (प्रत्याहार), dharana (धारणा), dhyana (ध्यान), samadhi (समाधि)

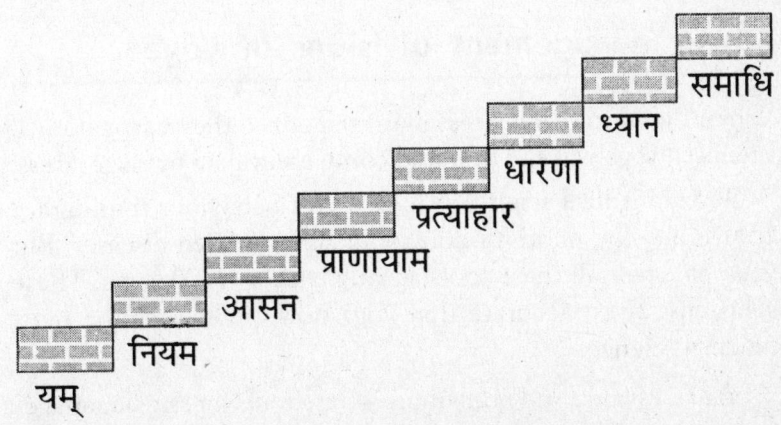

यम् -	Restraints and controls	
	Non-violence	अहिंसा
	Truth	सत्य
	Non-stealing	अस्तेय
	Celibacy and self-restraint	अहिंसा
	Non-hoarding	अपरिग्रह
नियम	Observations	
	Purity, cleanliness	शौच
	Satisfaction	सन्तोष
	Devotion to God	तपस्
	Self-learning	स्वाध्याय
	Dedication	प्रणिधान

आसन - Physical holds

प्राणायाम - Control of breathing

प्रत्याहार - Negation of hunger; control over senses

धारणा - Concentration; fixation of mind

ध्यान - Contemplation; flow of concentration, meditation

समाधि - Ultimate knowledge and control over all body functions and mind.

Stress management divisions of yoga

When I used to teach stress management to the heart patients, I realised yoga was the best and complete way to manage stress.

Today medical science is looking for behaviour training for controlling the mind for control of stress related diseases. But yoga has spelt all these tools as long back as 3000 years. These solutions are so accurate that yoga now qualifies as the most modern science.

Yama, niyama and pratyahara — are tools for stress management. They may be modified a bit to suit the modern conditions. When I teach yoga — I believe stress management is the best part of yogic advice. I am in the process of writing a complete book on yoga and stress management.

Meditation and pranayama are also very useful for stress management. They calm the mind and relax the body. They help in controlling the emotions.

Physical postures and yoga stretches

Yoga postures and stretches are useful for heart patients and are completely safe. They are exercises which tone the body, stabilise the mind and massage the internal organs without causing any angina and pressure on the heart. To me yoga is the best form of exercise that a heart patient can do.

We have selected some particular postures and stretches especially for coronary heart disease patients after considering them very scientifically. These asanas can be grouped into two broad categories:

A. HRE (health rejuvenating exercises)

B. Yogasanas for the heart.

In the next few pages we are going to explain how to perform them. HRE is very safe for severe diseases also but some of the yogasanas are to be restricted for heart patients. It is based on the clinical assessment investigations of the patients.

Health rejuvenating exercises (HRE)

These few posture movements mentioned below are preparatory to beginning the next step i.e. asanas. These are to be practised before beginning the yogic training.

    I. For the eyes

   II. For the neck

  III. For the ears

  IV. For the face

   V. For the shoulders

  VI. For the chest

 VII. For the waist

VIII. For the thighs and hips

  IX. For the knees

   X. For the ankles

  XI. For the toes and heels

I. For the eyes

A. Position

Stand at ease.

B. Movements

1. Keeping the head steady look up and down a few times.
2. Then look to your right and left, and further rotate your eyeballs. Try to cover a maximum range of vision.
3. Rub your palms to warm them and then put them over both your eyes and blink a few times.

II. For the neck

A. Position

Stand at ease.

B. Movements

1. Rub your palms together vigorously for 10 counts and

rub the back of the neck alternatively.

2. Repeat the same for the front 5 times.

3. Bend your neck backwards as much as possible and then touch your chin to the chest by bending forward. Repeat this 5 times.

4. Turn your neck thoroughly from the left side over the shoulders and vice-versa.

5. Bend your neck alternatively to both sides. Try to touch the ears to the left and right shoulders alternately.

6. Rotate the neck starting with the chin, touching the chest with the eyes closed, turn to the right with the eyes opened, ears touching the shoulders and further through the back looking up and left ear touching the left shoulder and back to chin with eyes closed. Do it on the other side also (2 rounds).

III. For the ears

A. Position

As above. Hold the upper portion of both the ears with the thumb and index fingers.

B. Movement

1. Pull both ears.

2. Pull straight out of the middle portion.

3. Pull down the lower lobes.

4. Cover both the ears completely with the palms, press and relax without taking away the hands to create vacuum in ears.

5. Make a fist with three fingers and thumb, leaving the

index finger free. Now with the index fingers rub the front of the ears.

6. With the same fingers now rub the back side of the ears.

IV. For the face

A. Position

Stand at ease.

B. Movements

1. Rub your face gently using both the palms.

2. Feel relaxed.

V. For the shoulders

A. **Position**

Stand at ease.

B. **Movement**

1. Keep your arms hanging straight down by your sides with fists closed. Raise the shoulders up, while inhaling and bring down while exhaling, without bending the elbows.

2. Rotate the shoulders backward to forward keeping the arms relaxed and repeat it forward to backward also (5 times each).

3. Bend your arms, fingers and thumb together touching the shoulders. Inhale and rotate the arms forward to backward and then backward to forward, while exhaling.

VI. For the chest

A. **Position**

Bend both the arms inwards, bringing the palms over the chest, facing it, with middle fingers meeting at the middle of the sternum.

B. Movement

1. Inhale and extend left hand, exhale and bring it to its former position. Repeat the exercise with the right hand (5 times each) and then do it with both the arms 5 times.

2. Keep your hands on the thighs. Inhale and raise the left arm touching the ear without bending, bring arms down and exhale. Repeat it with the right arm and then both arms simultaneously 5 times.

VII. For the waist

A. Position

1. Keep the feet apart as per the shoulder width. Arms should be hanging down by the sides of the body.

B. Movement

1. Raise the hands while inhaling, bend at the waist about 30° or more to the left while exhaling, bring left hand near the knee, bend neck to the left, drop the left hand also over the head, inhale and exhale 3 times. Reverse the process and come to the normal posture. Repeat this on the right side (2 rounds).

2. Lock the fingers and raise your hands.

   a) Turn palm upwards towards the sky.

   b) Bend at waist 30° or more to the left, arms straight with ears towards the left.

   c) Return to the position 1.

   d) Bring the arms down, repeat it to the right (2 rounds).

3. Keep palms together.

   a) Inhale and raise the hands upwards, arms straight

touching the ears.

b) Exhale and bend 30° or more to the left. (Inhale and exhale 5 times)

c) Return to position a).

d) Bring the arms down, repeat it to the right.

4. a) Inhale, raise the arms to the shoulder height apart at chest level, keeping the palms facing each other.

b) Twist at the waist so that the right hand goes to the left shoulder and left hand to the right hip. (Inhale and exhale 5 times).

c) Inhale and come to position a).

d) Exhale and bring the hands down and repeat the same on the right side (3 rounds).

VIII. For the thighs and hips

A. Position

Stand straight, keep the legs apart about 15 to 20 cms.

B. Movement

Strike the buttocks with the heel; alternately.

IX. For the knees

A. Position:

Keep the above standing position.

B. Movement

1. Let your left heel hit the hip; then stretch forward feeling a jerk at the knee. Do it with the right leg also. Repeat it 5 times.

2. Place your hands on the waist keeping your thumbs in the front. Keep both feet 30 cms apart. Keep the body

straight and bend knees as low as possible, then come up. Repeat this 5 times.

X. For the ankle joints

Raise the left leg a little above the ground. Move the ankle up and down 5 times. Then rotate from the ankle first clockwise and then anti-clockwise. Repeat it with the right leg also.

XI. For the toes and heels

Walk forwards on your toes, then walk backwards on your heels.

Yogasanas for the heart

Standing Postures

1. *Tadasana*

Position

Keep both heels and toes parallel and 10 cms apart; arms by the side.

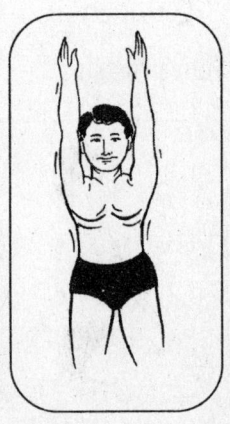

Movement

Inhale. Raise the arms up expanding the chest and abdomen slowly. Put back side of palms together, raise body on the toes. Hold the posture looking at a point at the eye-level. Keep the knees straight, bring the heels and arms down while exhaling as in the starting position.

Caution

Persons with slipped disc should not do this asana.

2. Padahastasana

Position

Stand erect with both feet together.

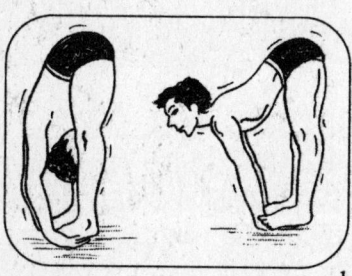

Movement

Raise arms, palms facing forwards over the head while inhaling. Exhale slowly while you bend forward, bring the palms down to hold the ankles and touch forehead to the knees. Try to keep knees and ankles straight. While you bend your body up to the level where you can bend easily keep in mind that the goal is to touch forehead to knees. Slowly raise your body while inhaling and taking arms up, exhale and bring the arms down.

Caution

The persons with a slipped disc (disc prolapse) should not do this asana.

Sitting Postures

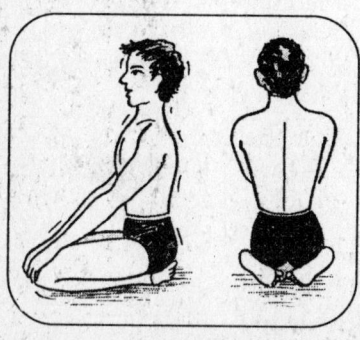

3. Vajrasana

Position

Kneel down.

Movement

Assume a kneeling position, heels open and apart and toes together, soles upward. Sit on the soles, keeping knees together. Inhale and exhale slowly and rhythmically.

4. Shasanksana

Position

Sit in Vajrasana posture and put palms together on the knees, keeping both arms straight.

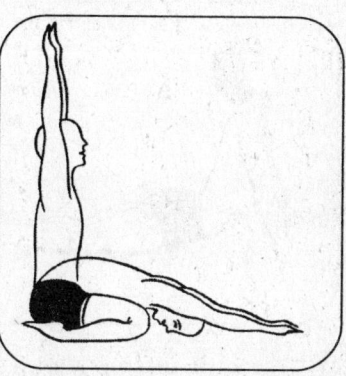

Movement

Inhale and raise joined arms over the head. Ensure that the arms touch the ears. Exhale and bend forward touching the floor with the palms. Inhale and exhale and maintain this posture for 5 breaths. Inhale and raise the arms along with the head. Exhale and bring the hands down. Do it twice.

5. Ardhamatshyendrasana

Position

Sit on the floor with both legs stretched straight in front.

Movement

Raise the right leg a little and bend the left leg and let the heel touch the right hip. Put the right leg and foot by the outer side of the left knee, sole on the floor. Bring the left armpit over the right knee. Hold the right ankle

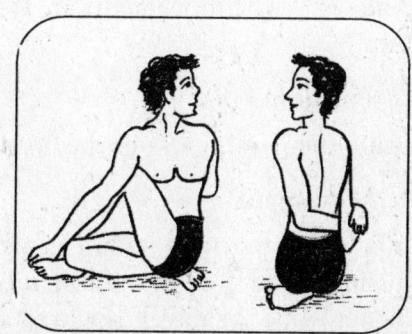

with your left hand. Exhale and stretch the right arm and swing back to touch the navel. Breathe evenly and maintain this posture for half a minute. Inhale and bring the right arm to the right side, exhale and free left hand and legs. Repeat this on the other side.

Lying Down on Chest Postures

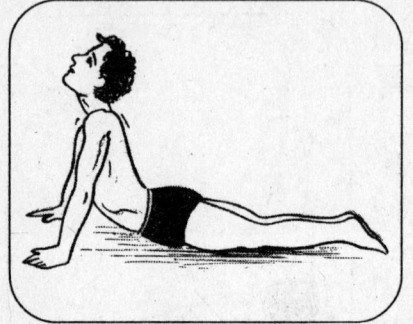

6. Modified Bhujangasana

Position 1

Lie face down keeping heels and toes together. Place palms about 30 cms apart from the body.

Movement

Inhale and come up 15 cms. Exhale with hissing sound from the mouth, pulling the navel inside. Inhale and raise the trunk on the palms and thighs and look skywards; slowly exhale with hissing sound and bring down the trunk to the floor.

Position 2

Bring the hands near to the body by about 15 cms.

Movement

The rest of the movements are the same as that of the 1st position.

Position 3

Bring the hands close to the body.

Movement

Inhale and raise the body 15 cms above the floor. Exhale with hissing sound from the mouth. Inhale and raise the trunk a little higher while the navel should touch the floor. Exhale with hissing sound and bring down the trunk on the floor. Spread hands beyond head on the right side of the face, keeping the toes together and heels open, relax the whole body. Turn the face and relax.

7. *Shalabhasana*

Position 1

Lie down on your chest with arms parallel to the body and chin on the ground.

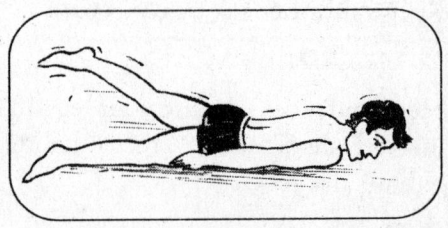

Movement

1. Inhale, turn toes inward, heels high, exhale, make the body stiff and raise right leg up from the floor as high as you can. Hold, inhale and exhale for one minute. Inhale and bring down the leg on the floor slowly and exhale.

2. Repeat with the other leg.

3. Now repeat with both the legs.

Lying Down on the Back Asanas

8. *Uttanpadasana*

Position

Lie down on your back keeping the fingers locked together, under your neck, and elbows on the ground. Keep both the feet 15 cms apart. You can also keep the hands parallel to the body.

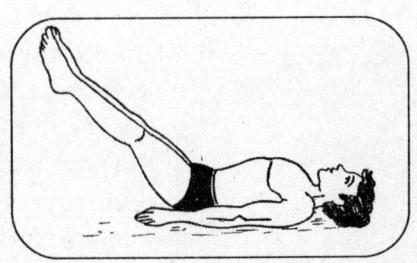

Movement

Inhale and exhale and raise both the legs 15 cms high above the floor. Inhale and exhale 5 times (inhale and bring your legs down and then exhale).

Position 2

Keep both the legs 25 cms apart.

Movement

Heels out, toes in, raise your legs 15 cms above the floor. Inhale and exhale 5 times. While inhaling, bring your legs down and exhale and relax.

Position 3

Keep your legs 45 cms apart.

Movement

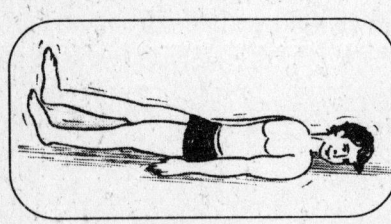

Do the same set of movements. Relax.

9. Merudandasana

Lie on your back with arms stretched at right angles to the trunk. Lift the left heel and put it on the right foot in the space between the big toe and the second finger, thus keeping your feet straight one above the other. Now stretch and rotate the upper part of the body (head and neck) towards the left and the lower parts (waist, thighs and

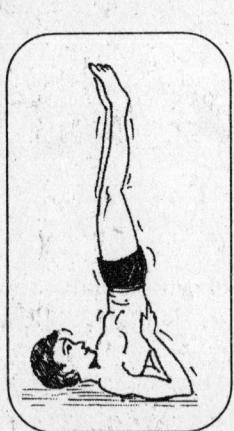

feet) towards the right while you inhale. The left toe should now touch the ground and the arms and shoulders remain in the same position as before. Now come back to the original position while you exhale. Now repeat the same on the other side.

Repeat the whole exercise after changing the leg position (Right heel over the left foot).

10. Sarwangasana

Lie down flat on the floor on your back with

legs stretched. Pull the chin inside and keep hands by side, palms facing the floor. Exhale and raise your legs to 90° taking care not to bend them at the knees. Exhale and raise the legs a little up and supported by the hands raise the whole body on back side of the head, shoulders and elbows. Try to keep the body straight. This is the complete posture. Slowly breathe a few times.

Follow the reverse steps in the same order and bring the body down slowly without any jerks. Relax.

Some More Asanas

1. Matsyasana

Sit in the lotus posture. Lie down on the back, raise the trunk with the help of elbows and head (on the ground). Hold both the toes with the hands. Let the arched trunk rest on the head and buttocks.

2. Ardha-Matsyasana

Those who are unable to perform Matsyasana, can practice this asana. Instead of assuming the lotus posture, spread the legs and with the help of the elbows raise the body up and bend the neck backwards; touch the head on the ground and hands on thighs. With the help of the elbows keep the head straight and relax.

3. Dhanush Banasana (Bow and Arrow)

Position

Lie with your face down, and arms and legs fully spread keeping them straight; toes and heels together.

Movement

Inhale then exhale; bend your left leg and hold it with the left hand and raise both the legs and arms above the floor. Keep this position for 5 breaths. Exhale and bring the legs and the arms in starting position. Do it with the right leg and then with both the legs.

4. Paschimottanasana

Position

Sit on the ground and stretch your legs forward. The toes are to be stretched away from the body as far as possible.

Movement

Now raise your arms straight up towards the sky, slowly beyond the head while inhaling. The palms should be facing each other and arms touching the ears. Exhale and bring your hands down and try to catch hold of your big toes with the index fingers. When you are able to do this pull the heels with your hands and place your elbows on the ground. Try to touch the knees with your forehead without raising the knees from the ground. Repeat this 2 to 3 times.

5. Pawan Muktasana

Position

Lie on your back keeping both the arms alongside of the body.

Movement

Stretch both the legs. Leaving the left leg on the ground, bend the right leg at the knee and bring the knee near the chest. Now inhale and press the bent leg to the chest with both arms, locked for this purpose. Keep the breath full in the abdomen and go on pressing the leg on it. Now, while exhaling, lift the head and try to touch the chin with the right knee. Inhale and bring the head back into normal position; and then bring the leg down and exhale. Repeat this with the right leg, and then with both the legs simultaneously.

6. Sun Salutation (Surya Namaskar)

This is a combination of seven yoga postures in a sequence of sixteen movements.

Position

Stand erect with the feet together. Place folded hands on your chest touching the Adam's apple with your thumbs and bend the head a little so that the index fingers are touching the centre of the forehead (Jyoti Kendra).

Movement No. 1: Inhale, raise the arms straight above the head touching the ears. Exhale.

Movement No. 2: Inhale and raise your arms vertically in line with the shoulders.

Movement No. 3: With both feet firmly on the ground keeping the body upto the waist erect, bend the upper portion of the body backwards.

Movement No. 4: Bring the arms together touching the ears, above the head.

Movement No. 5: Bend forward exhaling and try to touch forehead to knees placing both the palms by the side of the feet on the floor. Knees should be kept straight, while pulling the stomach inside.

Movement No. 6: Inhale and stretch the left leg backwards keeping the hands on the floor in the same position.

Movement No. 7: Bend forward and touch the floor with the forehead, while you exhale.

Movement No. 8: Inhale and raise your head upwards and look towards the sky.

Movement No. 9: Spread your right leg along with the left leg and keep the body parallel to the floor, toes and hands supporting the body during this.

Movement No. 10: Keeping palms and toes where they are, inhale, bend your arms and lower the body towards the ground touching only the forehead, chest and the knees on the ground. The buttocks should be kept high. Exhale.

Movement No. 11: Inhale. Raise the body on the palms and toes bringing the pelvis to the floor looking upwards at the sky while holding your breath.

Movement No. 12: Exhale and lift the buttocks and bend the head in, to see the navel.

Movement No. 13: Bring the right leg in between the hands and bend forward to touch the ground with your forehead.

Movement No. 14: Inhale and raise trunk looking up towards the sky.

Movement No. 15: Bring the left leg along with the right leg, head touching the knees as in posture No. 5, keeping hands by the side of the feet, fully exhale.

Movement No. 16: Inhale and stand up, palms together on the chest as in the starting position (2 rounds). Lie down and relax your whole body.

Yogic theory of diet

Under the yogic system, diet is classified as satvik, rajsik and tamsik. For people with coronary heart diseases, the satvik system of diet is the best. The Satvik diet has all the cereals, dals, fruits and vegetables which are in very close association with nature. Although milk and curd are also a part of the satvic food, the SAAOL Heart Program reduces their consumption to a minimal permissible amount, which is essential for the reversal of the blockages in the coronary arteries, as we shall see later. The diet should be fat-free and with no cholesterol, as far as possible. The intake of white sugar and salt should be moderate. Tea and coffee, or other caffeine containing beverages should be avoided.

Diet should be such that it has a considerable quantity of roughage. The covering (husks) of all grains, legumes, vegetables and fruits are rich in fibre contents and they also have some minerals, enzymes and antioxidants which are extremely essential for reducing cholesterol level in the blood.

An Ideal Daily Intake should be as Follows

Breakfast: Fruits, a bowl of dalia made of oat-bran, whole wheat, maize, millets and sprouts.

Lunch: Roti or chapati (preferably made of whole wheat, gram and soya flour), vegetable salads, dal, chatni, rice and soups. Atta 50% wheat, 25% soya and 25% Bengal gram).

Afternoon: Fruits and herbal tea.

Dinner: Dalia, khichari, kari, boiled leafy vegetables, sprouted and steamed grams like chick-peas (Bengal gram), moong, beans etc. Chapatis can also be taken.

Kayotsarga — progressive relaxation

This is an important practice of Preksha Dhyana. The literal meaning is 'to abandon the body'. '*Kaya*' means '*body*', and '*Utsarga*' means 'to drop or abandon'. In practice it is conscious suspension of all the gross movements of the body. The result is relaxation of the muscles and reduction of metabolic activities. This physical condition helps in relieving mental stress. Physically it is more restful than sleep and is most harmless and a direct antidote to psychosomatic maladies resulting from stress and anxiety. Gradually all the muscles are relaxed.

The Technique

This exercise can be done in any posture such as sitting, standing or lying down. When we practice meditation, it is essential that it is done while sitting. When we want to be free from tension, this is to be done while lying down.

The Pledge

The pledge is to be recited in the standing position. "I want to be free from my physical, mental and emotional tensions, for that I practice Kayotsarga. I pledge that I will maintain awareness throughout the practice." Lock the hands and give tension to the whole body by stretching it upwards raising the body on the toes and feel the tension in every muscle.

Step: 1

Sit or lie down keeping the spine and neck straight but without stiffness, eyes softly closed. Relax all the muscles of the body and let them become limp.

Step: 2

Focus your attention on each part of the body one by one. Allow each part to relax by auto-suggestion and feel that it has become relaxed.

Step: 3

For deep relaxation of the body and mind start with the big toe of the right foot; suggest muscles and nerves to relax, feel it relaxed and move on to the other part of the right leg — toes, sole, heel, ankle, calf muscles, knee, thigh, and buttocks. In the same way relax the left leg.

Step: 4

Relax the trunk from the hip-joint to the neck, starting with the back and front of the lower abdomen, upper abdomen, ribs, front and back, the chest muscles, collar bone and neck muscles. Then relax the right hand starting with the finger tips upto the shoulder, then the left hand from the finger tips to the shoulder joint.

Step: 5

Relax the upper part of the body from neck to head and throat, chin, jaws, lips, tongue, mouth, cheeks, nose, eyes, ears, temples, forehead, and scalp.

Step: 6

Feel and experience that the whole body is completely relaxed. When the body and mind are relaxed, remain in this condition for a few minutes.

Step: 7

Perceive the whole body to relax and feel it physically, mentally and emotionally relaxed. If there is any tension in any part, relax and once again feel the whole body totally relaxed. Maintain this posture for a few minutes.

Step: 8

To finish Kayotsarga, the body has to be charged with energy part by part, inhaling fully into each part. Start with the upper part of the head, face and neck, the middle part of the trunk, the right hand, then the left hand, the right leg and the left leg. The whole body! Inhale and turn to the left side placing the elbows below the neck. Slowly sit up. Take two or three deep breaths.

Pranayama

Nadi-Shodhan Pranayama

Sit in a comfortable posture and breathe normally. Close your right nostril with your thumb and inhale slowly through the left nostril. When the inhalation is complete, close the left nostril also and hold your breath for 2-3 seconds. Now lift the thumb from the right nostril and slowly exhale keeping the left nostril closed. Repeat the process by inhaling through the left nostril and exhaling through the right nostril. This is one cycle of Nadi-shodhan pranayama. Repeat this for 10 cycles.

Preksha meditation

Preksha Dhyana

This system of meditation is based on the wisdom of ancient philosophy and modern scientific concepts. Meditation does not mean suppression of mental functions. The main aim of Preksha Dhyana is to purify the mental state. When the mind is clean, peace of mind automatically surfaces. Balance of mind, equanimity and the state of well-being are experienced simultaneously.

Preksha means 'Perception' and Dhyana Meditation means 'Concentration'. So Preksha Dhyana means concentration of perception and not of thought. The mind is an instrument of thinking as well as perception. Perception is strictly concerned with the phenomena of the present. It is neither a memory of the past nor an imagination of future. Perception of the current happenings, must be a reality. In Preksha Dhyana, perception always means experiencing the benefits of qualities of likes and dislikes. In due course of time our conscious mind becomes sharpened to perceive internal realities. There are steps of perception to start with, and perception of breath is an important step in this system.

The mind freeing itself from the known is meditation. Meditation is the total denial of everything that the mind has accumulated. Meditation is the action of silence.

— KRISHNAMURTI

The Technique

Perception of Deep Breathing: Breathing is linked with the conscious mind. The mind is always restless, it is extremely difficult to steady the wandering mind directly. An efficient and easy way to control mental activities is concentrated perception of breath. At the same time, the rate of breathing can be reduced from 15-17 per minute to 10-12 per minute and by further practice to 4-6 per minute.

Step: 1

Do Kayotsarga, relax the whole body and feel it relaxed.

Step: 2

Direct your full attention to your breath, removing all thoughts and sensations. Regulate your breathing, make it slow, deep and rhythmic. Focus your attention on the navel and become fully aware of contraction and expansion of the abdomen accompanying exhalation and inhalation simultaneously.

Step: 3

Continuing the slow, deep and rhythmic breathing, shift your attention from the navel, and focus it inside the junction of the nostrils, from your attention on the process of respiration. Each and every inhalation and exhalation is to be perceived i.e. each and every breath is to be watched, felt and intentionally, consciously inhaled and exhaled.

Step: 4

If you are distracted return your attention to your breathing. If it is frequent, then hold your breath for a few seconds and then breathe again normally.

Step: 5

To finish meditation, take two or three long breaths. Exhale for three times and pay obeisance by bending forward.

Four Components of Meditation

Scientifically speaking all types of meditation have the same basic principles. Medical science has studied meditation in great detail. Hundred kinds of meditation are available today and people have asked me which one is the best. I feel all are good for the heart. Some are more focused on the heart.

The four basic components of every meditation are:

1. Quiet atmosphere/surroundings
2. Posture : Comfortable with spine straight and eyes closed
3. Passive attitude
4. Theme to follow.

Meditation: a scientific theory

Themes of Meditation

Earth elements	: Black dot, statue of God
Water elements	: River, lake, sea
Sound elements	: Word, mantra, japa, bhajan
Fire elements	: Lamp, candle
Nature elements	: Blue sky, dense forest, sun, moon, ice-peaks, sea waves
Body elements	: *Sharir* (organs), limbs, breathing
Psychic centres	: Kundalini
Colour	: Orange, green, white
Thoughts	: Anupreksha

What all is proved by now?

Medical research has already proved the effects of yoga, asana, meditation. Some of the important ones are as follows :

1. Blood pressure decreases
2. Pulse rate or heart rate decreases
3. Catecholamines decreases
4. Oxygen consumption decreases
5. Type-A starts becoming like Type-B
6. Anxiety level decreases
7. Flexibility increases
8. Serum cholesterol decreases
9. Blood glucose decreases (control on diabetes)
10. Smoking reduces
11. Physical fitness increases
12. Reduces sleeplessness
13. Better supply of oxygen in the lungs
14. Reversal of heart disease

Some practical tips about yoga

Total duration of the daily practice of yoga should be about 40 to 60 minutes. However, meditation can be practiced for longer periods, if one desires. The best time to practice yoga and relaxation is early morning, which is also very convenient for a regular practitioner or professional individual who has to go to work everyday. Ideally, the stomach should be empty. Some of the optimum requirements, other than these, are loose and comfortable clothes, quiet surroundings and an adequately ventilated room.

The training will consist of four separate sessions, each of 2 hours duration, where the patients along with their spouses will be taught all these procedures. They can, however, refer to the manual from time to time while they practice, as and when needed.

Rules and Regulations

1. Regularity and punctuality in practice is essential.

2. Time fixed for practice should be maintained. Early morning hours are ideal because the bowel is clean and the stomach is empty. For some people evening hours are also suitable. At least a 2 hour gap must be allowed between taking meals and practice.

3. A cup of coffee or tea or milk can be taken half an hour before practicing asanas, if one needs. Ideally avoid tea and coffee completely.

4. *Place:* Clean and airy place without noise or disturbance is ideal for asanas and experience.

5. *Dress:* Comfortable, loose and light dress is good for such practices.

6. *Sleep:* About 6 to 8 hours sleep is required daily for an adult. If one goes to bed early, it will be possible to have a sound sleep and to get up early in the morning. Only then it becomes possible to maintain proper timing for yoga practice.

7. *Rest:* While doing asanas if you feel tired, you should take rest. Please, never cross the limits of your capacity. The capacity increases slowly. After completion of the asanas, five minutes of Kayotsarg (muscular relaxation) is necessary. After that meditation can be practiced. Walk forwards on your toes, then walk backwards on your heels.

Anupreksha and moral code

Anupreksha means contemplation or reflection or thoughtful consideration. It can be done to get rid of many stressful aspects of our daily behaviour. Urges, impulses, emotions, passions can be controlled by it. It also teaches us a moral code. The total life-style can be changed to a more relaxed, stressfree and purposeful existence.

For heart patients, Anupreksha helps to open the blocked arteries. This practice of positive thinking has recently gained validation from medical science, and this latest branch of medical science is called psycho-neuro immunology (PNI). According to PNI, whenever positive thinking is done, positive neuro-chemicals are released in the body fulfilling our requirements or wishes. Dr. Dean Ornish has also used this procedure in his life-style heart trial for opening of the coronary arteries.

How to meditate for the heart?

Psycho-neuro immunology (PNI) is the latest branch of medical science. A huge amount of research findings now support that affecting the mind positively about any event, would lead to positive chemical secretions in the body. These chemicals would then work for the solution of the problem or event.

I recommend meditation for opening the blockages of the heart. If the patient thinks of opening the blockages in deep meditation the same would happen to him. The chemicals would be released and help in the removal of deposits.

SAAOL's meditation classes are held during the resort camps and some audio cassettes are available for this purpose. A meditation of minimum ten minutes daily is recommended.

A flash of green light is used during the meditation to open the heart. But first the patient has to relax completely. Usually Kayotsarg forms the first few minutes of meditation. I have adopted this meditation from Preksha meditation, as suggested by my Guruji Acharya Mahaprajna.

Role of Exercise

Contents

A healthy body is a guest chamber for the soul; a sick body is a prison.

— BACON

Lack of exercise —
the major cause of heart disease

With the advancement in technology, rapid mechanisation and economic prosperity, there has been a gradual drop of physical activity among people in all segments of the society. With the increased overload of work in the recent years, many people have given up exercise related activity in favour of other priority sectors like occupation, recreation, watching TV and so on. The body, which used to do much more physical activity does not now have to go for so much of the same, thus reducing its fat requirement in food. In the face of inactivity, whatever extra calories we consume, will keep on getting deposited in the body and in the arteries.

Think of a busy executive's life. He gets up at 7 am. Drinks tea, reads newspapers, talks on the phone, does some planning, takes a bath, has breakfast before leaving for office in a vehicle. In the office, he sits throughout, doing paper work, computer work and talks on the phone for long hours — all the time getting stressed. In the evening, he comes back by car, sits on the sofa to watch the TV, gossips on the phone, has a good meal and goes to sleep. The amount of exercise is practically nil. To reduce exercise further we have servants, a caring wife, remote control to change channels and a cordless phone.

> Exercise the heart and generally speaking, all parts of the body which have a function, if used in moderation and exercised in labours in which each is accustomed, thereby become healthy, well developed and age more slowly, but if left unused and idle they become liable to disease, defective in growth and age quickly.
>
> — Hippocrates, 300 BC

Such a person, has a fat rich diet with ghee, oil, cream (consider his calorie expenditure) which will definitely start depositing fat in the arteries.

One must remember that now low physical activity is very normal in urban life and food with meat, milk, ghee, oil and cream is never a normal diet for such a person. Diet has to change accordingly. The earlier normal diet is highly abnormal today. And if somebody chooses to adhere to this abnormal diet, he or she has to make sure that plenty of physical activity must also be part of their life. Otherwise heart disease, obesity, high blood pressure are not far away.

All parts of the body which have a function, if used in moderation and exercised in labours in which each is accustomed, become thereby healthy, well developed and age more slowly; but if misused and left idle — they become liable to disease, defective in growth and age quickly.

— Hippocrates

Exercise — a must for heart patients

The minimum number of times that the heart beats is about 70 times per minute (normal range 50 - 90), but it has a capacity to go as high as 200 beats. That is the maximum capacity that the heart can work in a normal young adult. But we do not allow the heart to work for more than 70 to 100 beats per minute. It loses its fitness and habit of reaching a higher sale and gradually capacity to work at high loads (while climbing stairs, jogging, fast walking, carrying heavy weight, running etc.) becomes difficult. This is called deconditioning of the heart. People having a de-conditioned heart get less breath and become tired even with slight physical exertion.

This deconditioning of the heart may prove more difficult if the arteries of the heart are blocked i.e. like in angina patients. On the slightest exertion the heart rate goes up and angina starts.

The requirement of the heart for a particular physical activity goes up tremendously.

This is the main reason why a heart patient must have regular physical activity. This makes the heart more fit, conditioned, active and resistant to angina.

Exercises are also useful because they burn calories, cut down the cholesterol, triglycerides and blood sugar levels. The following are the benefits of regular physical exercises.

Regular exercise is most pleasurable when it is part of your life's routine.
If you are not used to do strenuous exercise, walk-don't-run should be your motto at first.

— Voltaire

Benefits of exercise

Physical benefits

1. Enhancement of physical performance (ability to perform physical work without fatigue or strain on the heart)
2. Better control of angina
3. Better control of blood pressure
4. Reduced susceptibility to rhythm disturbances
5. Better control of body weight
6. Improvement in fat distribution
7. Greater efficiency of lung function
8. Better organ and limb circulation
9. Prevention of weakening of bones relating to age
10. Better cold and heat tolerance
11. Protection of joints
12. Reduced tendency to have hyperacidity

13. Better bowel function
14. Improved function and appearance of skin
15. Regression of coronary artery blockage
16. Reduction in recurrence rate of heart attacks
17. Increase in life-span.

Bio-chemical benefits

1. Reduction of low density cholesterol (bad cholesterol)
2. Increase in high density (good cholesterol)
3. Reduction in blood triglycerides (fat) levels
4. Better control of diabetes mellitus
5. Reduced risk for spontaneous clots
6. Reduction in stress induced, inappropriate, hormone secretions

Psychological benefits

1. Enhanced energy, enthusiasm and self image
2. Reduced anxiety and depression
3. Better ability to cope with stress
4. Better relaxation and sleep
5. Lower or no requirement of sleeping pills and drugs to control anxiety

Socio-economic benefits

1. Early return to gainful employment
2. Reduction in recurrent medical expenses

Health is a kind of fitness, a fitness for love, for work, for play, for thought — in short, a fitness for life itself.

— RICHARD B. GUNDERMAN

How much exercise is needed?

Normal Person

For a normal person there is no limit to exercise as there is no safety margin. They can go upto any limit that they prefer. The more they do, more they benefit from exercise. The minimum prescription of exercise for a healthy person is a brisk walk of at least half an hour. If they want to have very good physical fitness, trim body, lose weight, become an athlete or body builder they can go upto 2 hours daily. It is a common experience that people in the earlier days, regularly exercised or walked, had tremendous stamina and avoided heart disease even if they ate a lot of fat and meat.

Now, in modern times, exercise or physical activity has gone down tremendously. A normal person is advised a brisk walk for 30 minutes once a day, if he wants to prevent heart disease.

But one must remember that doing exercise to protect the heart does not allow one to eat plenty of meat, smoking or excessive stressful life.

Heart patients

Heart patients are under a tremendous dilemma when they are asked by doctors not to do exercise on one hand and perform regular exercises to keep the heart fit, on the other hand. When they exert beyond their capacity angina occurs. This gives them a fear of walking or to perform exercises, which is an absolute necessity for preventing blockage or reversing it. Due to lack of knowledge, many heart patients give up exercise and live a sedentary life. This, in turn, leads to aggravation of the disease.

Many cardiac surgeons and intervention physicians (those who perform angioplasty or stenting) unnecessarily scare the heart patients, not to carry on with any kind of exercise. This is often done with an intention to pressurise the patients to go for surgery or angioplasty. This has been a common practice now, due to rapid commercialisation of cardiac care.

There is absolutely no doubt that a heart patient needs adequate exercise to improve his heart condition. Only thing he should be aware of is the intensity of such activity or the duration. This needs a thorough understanding about the effect of exercise on the heart rate and the effect of heart rate on the production of symptoms.

Let me also admit that patients cannot do without a medically qualified doctor. By just reading the book his understanding will still be inferior to the physicians attending on him. Thus, getting advice from a cardiac rehabilitation physician cannot be undermined in this regard.

The rule of thumb is that the intensity of the exercise should be such that it does not lead to angina or symptoms of ischaemia in the patient. If increasing the walking speed or exercise leads to symptoms, the speed of exercise should be reduced. If walking is not possible due to angina (angina would mean chest pain choking sensation, breathlessness or other symptoms), it is advisable to increase the medicines (sorbitrate group) during exercise, heart rate goes up and along with the heart rate oxygen requirement of the heart also goes up. Till arteries are able to meet this increased demand and there is no deficiency, there will be no angina. Exercise till this stage is useful for the heart. The problem occurs only after the patient exceeds this limit. So, it is good to do a submaximal exercise for all heart patients. Which means maintaining a speed which does not create a problem.

The preservation of health is a duty. Few seem conscious that there is such a thing as physical morality.

— HERBERT SPENCER

How to calculate exercise intensity for a heart patient?

If someone wants a more scientific way of calculating the exercise intensity or speed, one needs a prior exercise stress test (or Tread Mill Test). As you will remember the theory of taking the test, the heart rate increased till the ECG shows shortage of oxygen. Exercise intensity is increased to increase the heart rate, through a motorised machine. The heart rate at which the ECG shows change is the maximum that a patient can safely reach. For an extra precaution, I would recommend 20 beats less than the Stress Test limit.

Another requirement for this process is that the patient should be able to count his own pulse rate at rest and during exercise or walking. This can be done by putting two fingers (index and middle) of one hand on the front of the wrist of the other hand and then counting the heart rate (same as pulse rate) with a watch. You should practise this at rest (when the heart rate is 70 or so per minute). Once the confidence comes, the same can be done while the patient stops suddenly after a walk and pulse can be counted for the first ten seconds. The actual heart rate during exercise can be calculated by multiplying by six. This rate should be twenty less than the heart rate reached during the exercise stress test.

Sexual activity and heart disease

Many heart patients give up all sexual activity in the fear that they may get a heart attack or angina. I feel this is not correct.

Heart patients are allowed sexual activity as it is a great reliever of stress. They must, however, stick to the following precautions:

1. Do not physically exert — be a passive partner as far as possible. Let the active part be played by the spouse.
2. Be gentle and keep a lot of time. Do not hurry up but enjoy.
3. A tablet of sub lingual sorbitrate can be taken, before the act of sex.
4. Slow down or stop whenever angina comes.

If you follow all the rules about food, exercise and yoga — you need not worry. You will be safe.

Follow-up of Heart Patients

Contents

Learning is not following

There is a huge difference between what we know and what we do. Reading a book, watching a health show on TV or gossiping about health or having a lot of theoretical knowledge about heart disease is not the end of the disease. Unless it is followed or adhered to thoroughly, the results will not be there.

I have seen many good cardiologists and physicians giving printed advice to patients, which never comes into practice. The charts that the dieticians give with the calorie limits and ticks on standard format are only followed for a short time. The same thing should not happen to this book, otherwise the results would not come.

If you know that a particular food item has oil and cholesterol and if you still consume it, nothing can help you in the treatment of heart disease. If your priority of reading newspapers or watching TV or relaxation prevails upon your exercise or walking time, exercise will always be neglected. These thirty minutes of yoga can save you from years of ill health.

If you buy this book and just leave it on the shelf to gather dust, please gift it to someone else who would use it. Of course, you may save the person from a major disease. But remember for yourself, you can only postpone your life-style treatment, but cannot avoid it. Once the disease aggravates, angina surfaces or emergency arises, you have to start following the real cure. Do not postpone your treatment. The 'treatment of heart disease' is not like 'time management' which, even if you don't do, it does not matter. It will definitely have dangerous consequences one day.

I have found many of my patients coming back to me after two bypass surgeries, two-three angioplasties or following a heart attack after living a wrong life-style within a few years of a by-pass surgery. That is no treatment in the real sense. Please do not fall in this category.

Ninety-nine percent of the failures come from people who have a habit of making excuses.

— George W. Carver

All components of the program are equally important

Heart patients already know and learn a lot about the precautions which are to be taken — yet they cannot get protection from heart attack or treatment, as from SAAOL. The reasons being, mostly, inadequate follow-up and knowledge. Knowledge should be total and they should follow all the instructions completely.

All the components of THE SAAOL Heart Program will lead to maximum control of all risk factors of heart disease and adherence to all the components of the diet would determine the results of the program.

The diet should be followed in all respects. If you do not eat meat, it is good for the heart, but if you still continue to have milk in a good quantity, it makes the program incomplete. If you still continue having almonds or nuts, after restricting the oil intake, you are reducing the success of the program. If you are following the no oil dictum, but still maintaining your over-weight status, it is a non adherence.

Same is the case for the stress management program. You should do both, Kayotsarga and meditation. Follow these regularly. Type A behaviour should be changed. Anger has to be controlled. The balancing of sectors of life should be done to reduce stress. Even if you have to join the practical three-day course of the SAAOL Heart Program, with your son or wife, you should do so. But please follow all sectors of the stress management program.

Exercise and regular walks are also very important parts of the program. Try to reach the sub-maximal exercise stage and walk at least half an hour daily. But do not exceed your limit.

Yogasana and health rejuvenating exercises (HRE) are very important parts of follow-up. It may take about 20-25 minutes every day, and should be done at least six days a week.

SAAOL is the most practical program

SAAOL or Science and Art of Living is the most practical program, tested all over the country on persons from all walks of life. It can be followed most practically, by a very busy executive, marketing person, housewife or retired person, young or old (we have seen many above the age of 80 years following the program very accurately) as well as by doctors, professors, advocates and businessmen. We have patients, who are very young and recently married, single without wife, villager without any hi-fi knowledge base and aggressive type-A persons. We have on our participants' list trained yoga masters, known spiritual heads, DM cardiologists, high profile — ever travelling businessmen — who have followed the program. Hard-core non-vegetarians, ghee eating Marwari Jains, (chain smokers, smoking 60 cigarettes a day), alcoholics, drug addicts, stubborn mothers-in-law, over punctual army personnel — all of them have been able to change their lives and improve their heart condition.

We have seen people travelling to 23 cities in 30 days, eating in the hotels everyday and still able to follow the program.

In the last 7 years since the inception of SAAOL Heart

Program — we have been able to treat more than 5000 people from every part of the country — North to South and East to West. Every city now, big or small, has a few SAAOL followers who have changed their lifestyle practically to follow the program. From Nepal, Bangladesh, Sri Lanka, every country of the gulf, South Africa, North America, Canada, Italy, Great Britain, Nigeria to the smallest villages of India, people have taken up the SAAOL way of life, proving that it can be followed to a great extent.

All our training components are based on practical life and real life situations. We have seen the follow-up growing with time as the improvement shows, after following the program. Not only patients but also their family members have adopted the program. Even people without any heart problem have found the program very useful. If thousands of people can do it, why can't you?

O Health! Health! the blessing of the rich! the riches of the poor! who can buy thee at too dear a rate, since there is no enjoying this world without thee.

— BEN JONSON

Long-term adherence

The good thing about the SAAOL Heart Program is that most of the teachings can be adhered to for a long time. Once the mind-set is clear after a practical follow-up, the patients have adhered to the program on their own, even after they got cured. Even after being completely off medicines and having the TMT negative, people found it good for following throughout their lives. Of course the vigorousness thereof can be reduced after you have reached your target.

I have a simple advice. Please follow the program, food, stress management as a medicine very strictly till you reverse your problem. Once you are normal, with all the risk factors completely under your control, angina completely controlled, you may reduce the strictness to some degree. By that time, maybe within one or two years, you will get used to the food habits, exercises and relaxations, you may not want to go back to your earlier lifestyle. Reverse till you are normal, then maintain status quo is the dictum.

Create an awareness around you

When you eat very tasty food without oil, it is not only healthy for your heart but it also makes you comfortable from your gas problems, obesity and so on. Not only will it reverse your heart disease, but also prevent its occurrence in your family, friends and relatives. I advise my patients to spread the SAAOL habits and create an awareness amongst others. This allows a better adherence, as the friends and relatives also get adjusted to the same food.

While following the SAAOL diet, I have come across two groups amongst our patients. One group feels very bad thinking they have been isolated. They avoid going to parties. Even if they go, they will not talk about this kind of zero-oil diet because people may laugh at their food habits. They follow the SAAOL food at home and do not talk about it to others. Though they enjoy what they eat, they do not create an awareness in their circle.

The second group is of those patients, who feel great about the food and wherever they go, they talk about the wonderful taste and the scientific advantages of this kind of very low fat, high fibre diet. If other people have doubts, patients invite them to their homes for dinner and serve them the same SAAOL food. Once friends and relatives find the food quality and taste equally good, there is an instant appreciation. They will further spread the message. An awareness is built up in this way and patients spread the popularity of SAAOL food, which suddenly becomes acceptable.

The same is true about HRE. Many friends and relatives of my patients now regularly do health rejuvenating exercises with great fondness and express their gratitude to them.

Fill up your own history sheet

Placed below is a proforma and the variables to be filled regularly, may be once in every 15 days.

Name : ———————————————————————

Age: ——————— Height: ——————— Weight:———

Optimum Weight according to chart:————

Target : ——————

Risk Factors
Non modifiable
1. Age
2. Sex : Male /Female after menopause
3. Heredity

Modifiable (definitely measurable)
1. Blood pressure : Ideal 120/80 mmHg
2. Blood (serum) cholesterol : Ideal 130 to 160 mg/dl
3. Blood triglycerides : Ideal 60 to 120 mg/dl
4. Blood HDL (good) cholesterol : Ideally more than 40mg/dl

5. Blood sugar fasting : Ideally 70 to 100 mg/dl

6. Blood Sugar PP (after food) Ideal 120 to 140 mg/dl

7. Body weight : Ideal

Modifiable (not definitely measurable)

8. Exercises : low/satisfactory/good

9. Stress : low/moderate/severe

10. Fibre intake : low/okay/good

11. Zero oil food : strictly done/few lapses/gross violation

12. Smoking/tobacco : nil/lapses

13. Alcohol: nil/once/more than once

14. Non-veg intake : nil/once/twice

15. Milk and milk products intake : within 200 ml of milk/ above.

Type-A Behaviour Scoring

SELF-ASSESSMENT OF TYPE-A BEHAVIOUR
(The glazer stress control lifestyle questionnaire

		1	2	3	4	5	6	7	
1.	Doesn't mind leaving things temporarily unfinished	☐	☐	☐	☐	☐	☐	☐	Must get things finished once started
2.	Calm and unhurried about appointments	☐	☐	☐	☐	☐	☐	☐	Never late for appointments
3.	Not competitive	☐	☐	☐	☐	☐	☐	☐	Highly competitive
4.	Listens well, lets others finish speaking	☐	☐	☐	☐	☐	☐	☐	Anticipates others in conversation
5.	Never in a hurry, even under pressure	☐	☐	☐	☐	☐	☐	☐	Always in a hurry
6.	Able to wait calmly	☐	☐	☐	☐	☐	☐	☐	Uneasy when waiting

7. Takes one thing at a time □□□□□□□ Tries to do more than one thing at a time, thinks about what to do next time

8. Slow and deliberate in speech □□□□□□□ Vigorous and forceful in speech (uses a lot of gestures)

9. Concerned with satisfying himself or herself, not others □□□□□□□ Wants recognition by others for a job well done

10. Does things slowly □□□□□□□ Does things quickly (eating, walking)

11. Expresses feelings openly □□□□□□□ Holds feelings inside

12. Has a large number of interests □□□□□□□ Few interests outside work

13. Satisfied with job □□□□□□□ Ambitious, wants quick advancement on job

14. Never sets own deadlines □□□□□□□ Often sets own deadlines

15. Feels limited responsibility □□□□□□□ Always feels responsible

16. Never judges things in terms of numbers □□□□□□□ Often judges performance in terms of numbers (how many, how much)

17. Casual about work □□□□□□□ Takes work very seriously (works on weekends, brings work home)

18. Not very precise □□□□□□□ Very precise (careful about details)

19. Tries to satisfy self □□□□□□□ Wants job recognition

20. Easygoing ☐☐☐☐☐☐☐ Hard driving

Your Total A/B Score = ☐

Scoring:

40 - 50	=	B2, relaxed and easygoing (Good)
51 - 60	=	Moderate Type-B, coping well
61 - 80	=	Neither Type-A nor type-B but a healthy AB
81 - 100	=	Moderate Type-A
101 - 140	=	Extreme Type-A, coronary-prone

Cardiac risk factor scoring

This special scoring is a comprehensive quantification of cardiac risk. It represents a cumulative risk of blockage. Lower the risk, more the chances of reversal. Please fill up the scores for yourself and find out where you are:

DESTINY	Your score

A. Male   - 10
   Female   - 5
   Female - 10	

B. Age
   More than 60 = 10
   50 - 59   = 8
   40 - 49   = 6
   30 - 39   = 4
   22 - 29 = 2	

C. Family History of CHD/High B.P./Diabetes
   Both Parents   = 20
   One of the Parents = 15
   Brothers/Sisters = 10
   Other Relatives = 8
   If CHD + HT`   = +2
   + DM = +2	

D. Place of Residence Big Metro = 20 Small Metro = 15 Town = 10 Village = 5		
E. 2 Years or more of Heart Disease = 20 High B.P. (H.T.) = 15 Diabetes (DM) = 15 Both HT, DM = 20		
F. Job/Profession Stressful = 20 Okay = 16 Low Stress = 10 Enjoyable = 5		

HABITS	Your score
A. Smoking or Tobacco Heavy > 30 = 20 Moderate 10 - 30 = 15 Mild 1 - 10 = 10 Past Smoker = 5 Non-Smoker = 0	
B. Alcohol Daily = 10 2 - 6 days/Week = 8 Once/Week or less = 6 No Alcohol = 0	
C. Vegetarian = 5 Non-Vegetarian = 15 Occasionally Non. Veg. = 10	
D. Oil Consumption/Day More than 10 Tsp = 20 5 - 10 Tsp = 15 Less = 10 Nil = 10	

E. Intake of			
Butter	=	3	
Cheese	=	3	
Ice-cream	=	3	
Chocolate	=	3	
Fast Food	=	3	

F. Regular Intake of (6-7 days)			
Salads	=	-10	
Sprouts	=	-5	
Fruits	=	-5	

G. Regular Fried Food Intake (6/7 days)			
Samosa, pakoda	=	4	
Burger	=	4	
Parat ha	=	4	
Puri	=	4	
Kachori	=	4	

H. Intake of Milk			
1 Litre/day	=	15	
500 - 990	=	10	
Below 500	=	5	
Skimmed Milk	=	-2	

PSYCHOLOGICAL	Your score
A. Type-A	
Score 100 + = 20	
70 - 90 = 15	
60 - 70 = 10	
Below 60 = 0	
B. Sector Analysis = Problems in	
Money = 5	
Work = 5	
Family = 5	
Love = 5	
Social = 5	
Spiritual = 5	
Hate = 5	

	Your score
C. Spouse Education/Work Professional = 5 Teacher /Clerical Job = 3 Housewife = 2	
D. Self Stress Scoring = 0 – 10	
E. Overload Analysis Work = 4 Time = 4 Information = 4 Requirement = 4 Illness = 4	
F. Family Interaction With Spouse = 5 Children = 5 Parents = 5 Others = 5	

ANTHROPOMETRICAL & MEDICAL	Your score
A. Weight +20 kg = 20 +10 kg = 10 +5 kg = 5	
B. Central Obesity Gross = 10 Less = 5 No = 0	
C. Skin Fold Thickness 10 mm plus = 10 5mm = 5 2mm = 2	
D. Blood Pressure Systolic > 200 = 20 140 – 200 = 10 120 – 140 = 5	

		Your score
Diastolic > 130	= 20	
100 – 129	= 15	
90	= 10	
80	= 5	
E. Physical Inactivity		
Walking > 5km/Day	= –10	
Walking 2 - 5 km	= –5	
<2 km	= 10	
Household or Less Physical Activity	= 15	
Almost no Physical Activity	= 20	
Yoga	= –5	

BIOCHEMICAL		Your score
A. Serum Cholesterol		
<150	= –5	
150 - 180	= 5	
180 - 200	= 10	
200 - 245	= 20	
> 245	= 30	
B. Serum Triglycerides		
<100	= 5	
100 - 160	= 10	
160 - 200	= 15	
>200	= 20	
C. HDL Cholesterol		
>50	= 5	
40 - 50	= 10	
30 - 39	= 15	
20 - 29	= 20	
D. Ratio		
<4	= 0 - 5	
4.0 - 4.9	= 5	
>5	= 10	

E.	Diabetes		
	Fasting > 120	= 10	
	100 - 120	= 6	
	<100	= 2	
	pp>200	= 10	
	150 - 199	= 6	
	< 150	= 4	
	< 120	= 2	
F.	LDL Cholesterol		
	> 200	= 10	
	150 - 199	= 5	
	130 - 149	= 3	
	60 - 129	= 2	

YOUR SCORE

	Your score
Destiny	
Habit	
Psychological	
Anthropometrical /Medical	
Biochemical	
Total	

RISK ANALYSIS

Score more than 400 (Very high risk)	=	100%
Score 200 - 400	=	(33 - 99%) Risk
Score till 200 (100-200 Reversal Range)	=	(First 33%) Okay
Score lower than 100	=	(0%) Almost no risk

Follow-up sheet

Name ....

SAAOL Code No. ....

Camp Date .... Place ....

MEDICINES

Medicine: Code and Dose

1.	7.
2.	8.
3.	9.
4.	10.
5.	11.
6.	12.

Date	Day	Morning	Noon	Evening	SOS	Remarks

Follow-up sheet

Name ....

SAAOL Code No. ....

Camp Date .... Place ....

YOGA AND DIET

DATE	DAY	PULSE RATE *	H.R.E. **	YOGASANA **	PREKSHA **	KAYOTSARGA **	DIET ***	WALK **

* per minute
** in minutes
*** whether restrictions followed or not

Note down whenever you go wrong

To err is human. Everybody makes a mistake knowingly or unknowingly. But once you have crossed your determined or already defined limits, to go back to normal, violate the rules only when it is absolutely unavoidable. Zero violation is not possible.

Even if you violate rules of the SAAOL Heart Program, please make a note of the same. Noting down in black and white always gives a sense of guilt and makes you adhere better in future.

I remember, I had a patient who refused to comply with my instructions to give up alcohol. He agreed that it is not good for the heart and health, and also agreed that a lot of people are still happy without consuming alcohol. He also agreed that he does not want his son, daughter or wife to start drinking. But he said he will still continue to drink. Since he was not under my control, I requested him to note down in the adherence column whenever he drinks alcohol. He just had to write "I had alcohol today," everyday he had alcohol, against the date in the adherence sheet. But he refused that too. He was shy to write that. Ultimately we agreed that he will put one star(*) in the column, whenever he had alcohol. He was also supposed to see me once in fifteen days.

When he visited me next, he was following the diet very strictly, but I saw 12 stars in his chart. Next time he visited, he had four stars. After about two months he did not have any star in his chart. He had left drinking completely. This is the purpose of writing down your non-compliance.

Sometimes I take a promise from a patient. If he breaks any rule he has to take punishment and also write down the fault. I told him whenever he breaks a rule he has to give up his favourite item for a day. This works very well. You may make a list of whatever you like doing in a day and decide what you would like to take as a punishment. It may be, not reading the newspaper, not applying perfume, not watching your favourite program on television.

Small stress reduction tip: Learn from mistakes and avoid negative self-talk.

Duties and responsibilities of the spouses and close relatives

Heart patients need a lot of cooperation from their spouses. As majority of the angina patients are male, their wives must be instructed to do a few things, which can immensely affect the outcome of the treatment. I have seen many wives give medicines from time to time, but that does not finish their responsibility. They can be of a greater help. Please go through the following points, to know what can be done by them:

1. Please take all possible education about heart disease. Go through this book thoroughly or attend courses offered by SAAOL. This knowledge would help both the husband and wife. At many places he may be going wrong and the wife can help rectify matters.

2. Take interest in the patient's follow-up, what he is eating; what he is doing and what should be done. Offer your suggestions. It will help him.

3. Try to eat the same food as served to the patient. It will make him happy and increase the adherence level. It will also help you to improve your health. I have seen many patients' wives only preparing food for their husbands. Though they themselves are over-weight, have high BP, still they do not follow the program. This is ridiculous.

4. Do not repeatedly criticize the patients for their mistakes

or point out their faults. This irritates them. Help them by gently pointing out their mistakes. Use communication skills, suggest and find out alternatives to rectify the problems. Repeated insults make the patients adamant and it hurts their ego.

5. Please accompany the patient for a walk. Once accompanied, they also feel cared for and satisfied. I have seen that many couples feel closer to each other psychologically by walking together. They talk about their problems, share views in privacy and be more attached to each other. Earlier they could not get so much time to talk to each other in their busy schedule.

6. If you also perform all the yogasanas, HRE and meditation along with your spouse (husband or wife), it is ideal.

7. Never create doubt and fear in the patient's mind. In case of doubt, read the relevant chapter of the book or talk to your doctor. Keep yourself cool and calm. Do not necessarily create worry and fear.

8. Insist on regular check-ups. The serum lipid profile test should be done every three months. Blood pressure is to be checked every few days if the patient has a history of high blood pressure. May be twice a week. Blood sugar is to be tested every fortnight in case of diabetic patients.

9. In the SAAOL Heart Program I recommend definite participation of spouses, relatives and even children.

10. Remember, patients are even more stressed and irritated than others. You may have to compromise with them a little more.

Small stress reduction tip: Over expectation is the enemy of pleasure.

11. In many cases, I have seen wives insisting on little oil, or pieces of meat or sweets to their husbands. They insist that this will make the bits of patients happy but remember these small bits of happiness can also be offered by talking nicely to them, accepting their comments, and taking better care of them etc. Don't insist on wrong food. Many wives do not know that this will harm their husbands no end.

12. Do not make negative comments: I have heard many comments like: " You are looking weak", "You look pale", "You look tired". Always make positive comments. Appreciate the patient's achievements.

13. When you serve food to the patient, please give a variety. Same food makes the diet monotonous. You may even give a set of dishes to the patients and ask them to choose. Think of new ideas to improve the taste of the food. Add chutneys and taste boosters.

14. Arrangement of salads on the plate and decoration on the dining table also whet the appetite and acceptance of the food. Please work on these aspects.

The secret of care of the patient is caring for the patient.

— FRANCIS PEABODY, M.D.

Parameters needed for reversal

A comparison of usual cardiology with SAAOL recommendations

Causative factors	Usual Cardiology recommendation	SAAOL recommendation
1. Serum cholesterol	130 - 200 mg/dl	130 mg/dl
2. Serum triglycerides	60 - 160 mg/dl	Less than 120 mg/dl
3. Serum HDL cholesterol	30 - 60 mg/dl	More than 40 mg/dl
4. Cholesterol: HDL Ratio	4 - 5	Below 4
5. Serum LDL cholesterol	30 - 130 mg/dl	Below 100 mg/dl
6. Blood pressure (systolic)	120 - 140 mmHg	120 mmHg or less
7. Blood pressure (diastolic)	70 - 90 mmHg	80 mmHg or less
8. Blood glucose (Fasting)	80 - 110 mg/dl	80 - 90 mg/dl
9. Blood glucose (PP)	120 - 160 mg/dl	110 - 130 mg/dl
10. Smoking/tobacco	To be reduced	Banned
11. Exercise/walk	Should be done	Must do, at least one hour
12. Weight	20 - 30% extra (from any chart)	Only 2 - 3 kg extra allowed/permitted from Indian chart
13. Fibre intake	Not specified	Plenty everyday
14. Stress	Not defined, not available	Clearly defined, optimal
15. Total fat intake	10 - 30% calories	10% of total calories
16. Visible-fat intake	PUFA, MUFA etc.	Banned
17. Cholesterol intake/day	Not defined	10 mg/day

Take care of the minutes, for hours will take care of themselves.

Happiness is within you

Everyone needs happiness. Food can also give happiness, but it is not certain. I have seen people who have all the foods at their disposal and are still unhappy. I have seen many people who have such wrong notions of happiness.

Once a patient asked me: "Doctor, you don't eat meat?" I said no. He opined, "Your life is 50% lost without meat. You can't enjoy your life at all." I was amused. He again asked, "Doctor, you don't take alcohol?" I said no. He immediately declared, "Your life is 75% gone." When he was told that I do not even smoke or have tea and coffee, he immediately remarked, "Your life is a waste — you should commit suicide!"

I was astonished by his ideas about enjoyment of life. I can easily see how happy I was compared to whatever his life was. Happiness is inside us. People are happy even with a dry piece of bread on the footpath and people are not happy with so much meat and ice-cream at home. Please change your attitude towards food, and every dish will taste delicious.

Some people choose strict rules and regulations for happiness and some break them. Some people marry for happiness, and for some marriage is the most important cause of unhappiness. You have to decide whether you want to be happy. The rules of stress management have been laid down in the previous chapters of the book. They are complete and applicable universally. Just try to understand them.

Happiness lies first of all in Health.

— George William

Create a heart disease free society

Heart disease is a man-made disease. It is a disease born out of ignorance. It exists because we have failed to understand stress and to create happiness. It is because we have neglected our health. I often try to think whether it is possible to create a society free from heart disease.

I have a lot of evidence that such a society is possible if proper awareness is created. In the last three decades, in Europe and America, there has been a decline in the number of heart patients. The number of bypass surgeries has gone down recently in the United States of America. All this happened as people learnt to eat proper food and exercise regularly. It will need a concerted and mass effort. There the food that is sold in the market has break-up of calories, saturated fat and cholesterol, so that people can choose for themselves. Vegetarianism is gradually becoming a fashion. Smoking is now recognised a step closer to drug dependence, and is banned in most public places.

SAAOL Heart Club and SAAOL family

SAAOL is now gradually spreading all over the country and abroad too. When the participants of SAAOL stay together during the three days they become almost like a family. Then they meet the older groups and get support from them and thus the family becomes bigger. Since all the participants of SAAOL alongwith their individual families meet from time to time, following the same principles in life with regard to food, stresses, yoga, walk and exercises – the concept of a bigger SAAOL family was thought of.

The most important thing which binds the SAAOL family together is the helpfulness of the members. They help each other without any expectation in return. They value each other by sharing views as a matter of pleasure. There is no exchange or demand in return for favours. The love sector thus grows stronger.

On the last day of the course of SAAOL, a get-together is arranged wherein SAAOL participants of the last three years are also invited. Many of them are present there as they love such group meetings. We are proud to say that today there are about 1500 units of SAAOL family all over the country. Many are now also in USA, Canada, West Indies, Nepal, Sri Lanka, South Africa, Nigeria, Kenya, England, Abu Dhábi, Muscat and Bahrain.

Let us try to define the SAAOL family now. Anyone who follows the broad principles of SAAOL — Science And Art of Living — anyone who more or less follows the diet advised by SAAOL, spends time on exercise, yoga and meditation and also follows stress management techniques accordingly, is a member of the SAAOL family. The members are ever growing.

With the advent of Heart Talk, books and literature on SAAOL, we further plan to expand the SAAOL family in future. I hope in the years to come SAAOL would be a name known all over India as well as the world.

I am a great believer in luck, and I find the harder I work the more I have of it.
— Stephen Leacock

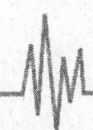

Section 13

Miscellaneous & Confidence Building

Contents

Comments by patients

On the occasion of the 2nd Annual Function, we had received lots of congratulatory mail from our old participants. We are reproducing a few below:

— SAAOL

I had angina on 27/1/97. Investigations revealed antroseptal myocardial infarction with normal LV function. Invasive investigation coronary artery angiogram revealed discreet eccentric lesion in proximal LAD with high takeoff of D_1, D_2 before 1st septal perforates. Doctors advised to have early revascularisation either CABG or angioplasty. In the meantime I joined the SAAOL Program on 25/4/97. I am continuing the diet (zero oil) — fat free vegetarian diet, regularly walking 4.9 kms/45 minutes, HRE and yogasana and Kayotsarg. I am feeling better, no anginal episode, I have reduced my weight from 77 kgs (Jan.) to 67 kgs (Sept.). I am very thankful to Dr. Bimal Chhajer. I wish him all the success in his program.

Dr. K. Udayakumar, MD, DM
Consultant Cardiologist, Villupuram, Tamil Nadu

An angina case with a strongly positive TMT, I suffered from acute breathing problem and could not walk even small distances without regular doses of sorbitrate. I joined the SAAOL Heart Program on 12th Jan. '96. But miraculously, during 4 days of hectic schedule of a balanced diet, yoga exercise, confidence building in self and the loving and serene atmosphere at the Suraj Kund camp, I did not take sorbitrate even once. Fortified in my resolve, the first thing that I did after reaching home was to throw away the sorbitrates in the dustbin, and happily enough there is no looking back since then. Having followed the diet, yoga and HRE exercises religiously for the last 20 months, now I neither experience any difficulty in breathing nor any chest pain. My TMT which was strongly positive will become negative soon, the quantum of medicines has been halved. There is a decrease in weight by 7 kgs

> Every day, in every way, I am getting better and better.
>
> *— ÉMILE COUÉ*

and I can walk for miles without any breathing problem. Today at 65, I feel remarkably light and active with a renewed hope and confidence that soon I will be totally cured from my heart disease. All the credit for this goes to Dr. Bimal Chhajer, I fail to find appropriate words to express my gratitude to him.

V.P. Kapur

Retd. Govt. Official and Poet, New Delhi

Angiography tests at AIIMS in July, 1995 showed 3 arteries blocked. As such I was advised bypass surgery. In the meantime I contacted Dr. Bimal Chhajer and joined his SAAOL Heart Program in September '95 in the 1st Batch at Suraj Kund. The program was so nicely managed, that it impressed me at the first instance. I followed the program which has completely changed my life-style and got rid of the disease. Since then I have had no problem. I took refund of my money which was deposited at AIIMS after a few months. Now after 2 years I am perfectly alright and am following SAAOL comfortably.

It gives me pleasure to record that the SAAOL Program has bypassed the bypass surgery. My TMT Test in May 1996 was 9 minutes. I am highly thankful to Dr. Bimal Chhajer and his staff for their kind cooperation and advice from time to time.

I wish the SAAOL Heart Program every success.

S.B. Sharma

Retired Executive, Faridabad

I was waiting for bypass surgery at bed No. 411 (7-12-95 to 20-12-95), Escorts Heart Institute, Delhi. I was informed by a fellow patient about SAAOL. I contacted Dr. Bimal Chajjer on the phone. Assured by the veracity of claims made by SAAOL, I got myself discharged from Escorts and joined Dr. Chhajer's Camp on 12-1-96. Doctors at Escorts told me that I ran the risk of heart attack any moment, but SAAOL has taught me that adherence to its program not only rules out any further deterioration of the heart but also improves its functioning. I am happy that I have improved a lot since then. My initial apprehensions about the efficacy of this program proved totally false. Before joining the camp I could not walk even 100 yards. It's about two years since I joined SAAOL. Now I walk 3-4 kms. daily in the morning and in the evening. I work 5-6 hours a day to honour my academic commitments without any trouble.

Medicine mingled with the philosophy of living advocated by SAAOL is a million dollar prescription for heart patients.

> Small stress reduction tip: Over perfection is a never-ending game.

Nobility has a nest in the nature of Dr. Chhajer and sincerity has a seat in the soul of every member of his team.

Dr. Raghunath Airi
Sanskrit Scholar, Gurgaon, Haryana

I along with my wife attended SAAOL Heart Program about a year back at Suraj Kund. During the last one year I have tried to religiously follow what was taught to us in the program. Since then I have not had any problem and am leading a normal life. Thanks to SAAOL, like me many other heart patients have been benefited by this program. We have been saved from avoidable angioplasty and heart surgery by following the SAAOL Heart Program. I decided not to go for them even if my company would pay for it. I wish SAAOL would grow and benefit heart patients throughout the length and breadth of India.

Y. P. Sabharwal
Govt. Executive, New Delhi

Since my bypass surgery in July 1989, I had never felt comfortable and was living with the usual fear, anxieties and worries which invariably catch people with heart disease.

But after spending 3 days with the SAAOL Heart Centre in March 1996 and thereafter, following the life-style taught by the centre for about one and a half years now, I find myself a totally changed man. Even my near and dear ones see the difference for the 'GOOD'. I think it has been a wonderful thing that has happened to me in joining and learning the Art Of Living with the heart disease at the SAAOL Heart Centre. I must admit that I probably follow only 70% of the program and the benefits are immense. Such things can at best be described only in person though. I wish more and more people, not only heart patients, but others as well, also get to know of such programs and adopt them early in life to lead a life of joy and happiness which is rare in the present environment.

My wife and I send our 'best wishes' to the SAAOL Heart Centre for its prosperity and in achieving more and more by doing such great service to the people. Regards!

Lt Cdr Rakesh Sharma
Naval Officer, New Delhi

I have participated in the SAAOL Yoga camp in June, '97 at Madras with L.V. disfunction suffering breathlessness, giddiness, palpitation and low pumping weak heart.

For the past 1 months I am slowly practising H.R.E, yoga, asana, pranayama, meditation, Kayotsarga and walking.

I am getting the following benefits by practising the SAAOL treatment regularly:

Before treatment	After treatment
1. Having giddiness regularly	Giddiness completely removed
2. Having palpitation, if strained	No palpitation felt
3. Unable to sit, walk, or eat more	Able to sit, walk, talk, eat more
4. More breathlessness	Breathlessness reduced
5. Tired life	Active life.

I am very thankful to Dr. Bimal Chhajer, for his SAAOL Camp. My weak heart is getting stronger and stronger. Please continue the SAAOL Heart Program all over India so that more heart patients would be benefited. Curing heart patients is a service to God. God Bless you and your family.

I. Danaseelan
District Chairman, Environmental Lions Club International
Paramakudi, Tamil Nadu

I had hypertension since 1964 when I was 28 years old. I am also a diabetic under treatment since 1972 and was on high dose of insulin. I got my bypass surgery done in 1991.

Since 1995, my treadmill tests again became positive and I also put on weight. I was 92 kgs. in January, 1997 in spite of walking and dieting. This was attributed to the high dosage -60 units of insulin I was taking.

I underwent the SAAOL Heart Program by the end of April, 1997. I was initiated into SAAOL exercises comprising health rejuvenating exercises, yogasanas and pranayama. The other yogic practices included were meditation and kayotsarga.

I also received valuable advice on diet and was initiated into the techniques of stress management. The importance of changes in life-style also impressed me.

Since then I have been following the diet and stress management principles very carefully. Due to some other health problems, I could not do the exercises 100% but still managed them on most days.

I have now decreased my weight by 7 kgs., feel much better and the occasional tightness in my chest has almost disappeared. My cardiologist has reduced medications and discontinued Nitrocontin totally. Now I take only 24 units of insulin per day.

I am sure with the momentum so far gained, over the next few months, I will be able to attain the targeted ideal weight and also make the treadmill test negative, in addition to discontinuing insulin totally.

I now have a sense of well-being, after starting the SAAOL Program and my quality of life has also improved both at home and in the office.

A. Krishnan
Ex. Managing Director, Cauveri Sugar and Chemicals Ltd., Tamil Nadu

What should I say about SAAOL Heart Centre. It is a God given gift for heart patients. I went to share my personal experience at one of the Program Sessions held in 1995. I had Angina trouble since December, 1993 and had to be admitted in M.P. Heart Centre, G.K. M.D. and on their advice I had an angiography test in G.B. Pant Hospital. Before that Test, the Echo and TMT were done but in Angiography Test, two blockages were observed in two different arteries i.e. 1st at 90% and 2nd 15%. I was worried as to how will I overcome this great problem. The doctor had suggested to get angioplasty first, if blockages reoccur then to have bypass surgery to remove blockages. Through some reference, I met Dr. Bimal Chhajer, Director/Chairman of the SAAOL Heart Centre for treatment of my angina trouble and as per his advice, I had undertaken Heart Care Program in 1995. After attending that course, I have been doing regular asanas/exercises/meditation, total control on diet. By doing all this, I controlled my weight/cholesterol etc. After that I have not experienced angina trouble again. I have not even touched sorbitrate tablets. Isn't it a "God given gift" through Dr. Chhajer and his entire team.

J.R. Nandwani,
Retd. Govt. Official, New Delhi

I am feeling a lot of improvement physically and mentally. I feel very confident and comfortable. After following the course of SAAOL Heart Program, I feel fit myself. I am very satisfied with your program. With this program I was able to reduce my medicines and weight as well. Before joining there was not so much of a strict routine program. Now with your guidance and ad-

> Only constant repetition will finally succeed in imprinting an idea on the memory of the crowd.

vice I am getting used to a normal routine. I have got so much satisfaction that I have encouraged others also to join your programme. Thank God and thanks to you that I am saved from medical treatment like bypass surgery etc. TMT is negative now.

Pardeep Kumar Arora
Govt. Official, New Delhi

I suffered a heart attack due to the tension of my wife's death and also eating fried things. Although I am a tee-totaller, yet I suffered a heart attack. I acted upon the advice of Dr. Bimal Chhajer, stopped fried things and tension. Now I am in good health. Thanks to SAAOL Heart Centre. There is a proverb, "Diet cures more than a doctor and as you sow, so shall you reap."

Dr. B.S. Bedi
Yoga Teacher, New Delhi

For the past four months, since 27th, April, 1997 there had been no, I repeat 'no' occurrence of any heart trouble in me. This event itself is a positive proof that the program I have been inducted into by SAAOL, and which program I follow diligently with ease, grace and convenience, is the only best medical attention one can have in conditions which I have been subjected to – viz., two vessel heart disease.

K.S. Krishnamurthy
Tamil Nadu

I have improved a lot after attending the course held at Mount View Hotel, Chandigarh, from 1/7/97 to 3/7/97. By changing the life-style, I have made a tremendous achievement in improving my health. I have made it a part and parcel of my life so that I may achieve further improvement.
I congratulate and wish all the best to SAAOL Heart Centre, Delhi.

R.L. Gaba
Bank Official, Chandigarh

I joined the course on 8th August, 1997 and I feel fresh from within and physically. I think that this program is very good. I am doing all the activities as I was told during the course. My views are that people who follow this program will definitely be all right.

Man Mohan Singh
Agriculturist, Meerut

By advocating a change in lifestyle, Dr. Chhajer at SAAOL Heart Program has conveyed to us that we can live on this earth without fear of death (because of heart problem) or we will say "अगर धरती पर स्वर्ग है तो यही है यही है।"

Ramesh Kumar Arora
Businessman, New Delhi

I suffered a heart attack in the year 1990, more than seven years back. I underwent angiography in 1993 and came to know that one artery was totally blocked and the second one was about 35-40% blocked. The condition continued to worsen and again angiography was done in July, 1996. The blockage of the second artery had increased to eighty per cent.

In the meantime I came across an advertisement in *The Hindustan Times* and contacted Dr. Chhajer. He assured me that there was no need of any angioplasty/surgery. I joined the program in October/November, 1996. Since the completion of the program, I can proudly say that I feel much better and the intake of sorbitrate has been considerably reduced. I am happy to say that I had to take sorbitrate only four times in a period of nine months.

I can boastfully say that the entire credit goes to SAAOL that I am keeping fit. I was so impressed that I became a member of the Heart Club and I am deriving benefits from the lectures being delivered by Dr. Chhajer.

With this I wish SAAOL a big success and I am of the firm conviction that this Centre will progress tremendously day-in and day-out.

R.K. Khurana
Retd. Govt. Official, New Delhi

I am 36 years old. I had a heart attack in September, 96 and had to undergo angioplasty in Apollo Hospital, Delhi by Dr. K.K. Saxena. But after angioplasty I was never confident and always felt very insecure. After joining the SAAOL Heart Program in April, 1997, I reduced about 5 kgs and felt quite energetic. I work 12 hours a day and now I am confident and feeling active.

Sanjay Jain
Businessman, New Delhi

I am a heart patient of two blocked arteries — one is 95% and the other is 65%. The doctor advised me to undergo coronary angioplasty immediately. Fortunately, I came in contact with Dr. Bimal Chhajer who is doing epoch making treatment no doubt.

I have the pleasure to inform you that as per the SAAOL Heart Program I benefited within a couple of weeks. Now I can walk 2-3 kms. at a stretch and I can go up the staircase to the 3rd floor without any fatigue. Now, I am thinking of reducing the medicine consumption if the doctor so advises me.

Manas Ranjan Kundu Chowdhury
Calcutta

I had angina and a positive T.M.T. report. My blood cholesterol report (lipid test) was also not in my favour. I was advised angiography by P.G.I., Chandigarh in February, 1997 which I kept postponing. I heard about the SAAOL Heart Program but frankly speaking I had reservations about its effectiveness. As luck would have it SAAOL arranged a camp at Chandigarh in the first week of August, 1997 and on persuasion of my family members, I participated in it. After six weeks, to my utter surprise and great relief, I found myself improving. Now I am leading a nearly normal life. I follow their instructions meticulously in my daily routine. Now I can walk for about 1½ kms without strain/heaviness in my chest. I hope to improve further as time rolls on. May SAAOL continue to lead in alleviating the suffering of the people having heart problems.

M.S. Chawla
Chandigarh

The SAAOL Heart Program is a very effective method of the reduction of the blockage in the arteries. It is based on nature cure. Diet control, yoga and meditation are the three main components of the treatment. Unlike angioplasty treatment and surgery etc, this system permanently cures the patients. I had attended the course between 9th August to 12th August, 1996. At that time I was in a very bad shape and doctors of G.B. Pant Hospital had advised me to get angioplasty done. After the treatment of SAAOL Heart Program I have reduced my weight by 24 kgs. Earlier my weight was 92 kgs. and now it is 68 kgs. which is normal. Now I am attending to my normal activities without any problem. I can assure you that this program has improved my health. I am very thankful to Dr. Bimal Chhajer and wish him all the best in his mission.

K.L. Chugh
New Delhi

I had blockage in two of the main arteries and was advised bypass surgery by doctors. Then I read about this Program. I joined Dr. Bimal Chhajer's SAAOL Heart Program at Khandala camp in Mumbai. In this program doctors treat various problems related to heart, stress, diet and meditation giving peace of mind.

At present, after 6 months of treatment, my problems are almost over. I am feeling quite normal. I feel that the SAAOL Program is very useful for heart patients.

Khatri Abdullah Sumar
Executive, Mumbai

Joining the SAAOL Heart Program has helped me a lot by improving the quality of my life. Earlier, I could barely walk 200 - 300 yards without getting breathless. Now I enjoy long walks both in the morning and evening. The medication for high blood pressure as well as diabetes have both been reduced and their control is more within the normal ranges than before. I am more scientifically aware of what I eat. I feel healthier in spirit and body now that I am doing regular yoga and other exercises. I am very grateful that Dr. Bimal Chhajer has come up with this venture.

T.D. Sethi
New Delhi

It has been a great experience to be associated with SAAOL Heart Program as a patient of coronary heart disease during September, 1996, which I will never forget. The recovery was amazingly fast.

After a break of nearly 3 months, I was able to resume my office work and activities. I am delighted to see that SAAOL has been growing and is completing 2 years of service in the treatment of heart disease.

Hearty congratulations to Dr. Bimal Chhajer and SAAOL on the completion of 2 years of exemplary service for which it was created!

Dr. R.K. Bhatnagar
Scientist, New Delhi

First let me wholeheartedly congratulate the SAAOL team for their excellent conduct of SAAOL Heart Program and sincerely wish them all success in their endeavours to bring forth new ideas for the program. In May, 1997, I had the first attack and underwent angiography for bypass surgery. On 16th June accidently I saw

> The distance doesn't matter; it is only the first step that is different.
> — MARQUISE DU DEFFAND

in the *Hindu* an advertisement about SAAOL Heart Program and attended the course from 20 - 22nd June, 1997 at the Taj Hotel. I have lost 10 kgs and can walk 7 kms/day without any problem. Thanks to SAAOL. Now I feel much better by strictly following the program. On this anniversary I wish you all the success.

V. Subramanian
Tamil Nadu

I had an acute myocardial infarction on 19th February, 1997 after an almost normal day at the office. I had the blood pressure reading of 90/40 and was put on Sorbitrates (3) Metoprotol (2), Envas (2) and Disprin (1). An angiogram was done and two blockages of 90% were diagnosed.

After attending the SAAOL Heart Program, during the 2nd program at Chennai (June '97), I followed the advice strictly with a lot of emphasis on walking and exercise. My cholesterol level dropped from 209 to 160, triglycerides dropped from 209 to 119, HDL and LDL from 37-40 to 43-93 and BP dropped to 110/80. Based on the above readings, doctor has advised me to stop the sorbitrates, since I feel comfortable doing normal routine work.

S. Balaji
Railway Official, Chennai

Firstly good wishes for the resounding success of SAAOL. Our congratulations are always there.

I am happy to be a member of the SAAOL family and have already benefited a lot. Have yet to undergo the lipid profile/TMT but I am rid of the symptoms and now happily walk around briskly including steep uphill in Shimla without angina or any problem(s) which were with me since 1983. A big THANKS. All the good wishes once again. Regards and God bless you.

Naresh Trehan
Shimla

My angina problem was detected in June, 1997 and I attended the SAAOL Heart Program held at Chandigarh from 1/8/97 to 3/8/97. Since then I have been following the dietary regimen and regular walk/yoga/meditation as advised in the SAAOL Heart Program. The positive indications of improvement started appearing after a period of one month. The giddiness and breathlessness have shown substantial downward trend and I can now go about my normal activities without any discomfort. Even otherwise, I have started feeling fit and healthier than before and I am confident that I shall recover fully within the next 2-3 months.

Brig. W.S. Choudhary (Retd.)
Panchkula

I was recommended the SAAOL Course by one of my friends who had joined the course previously. I joined SAAOL on 8th August, 1997. I feel myself, my wife and I have completely changed ourselves to the SAAOL styles and are extremely happy about it. When we weighed ourselves, I had lost 3 kgs. and my wife had lost 2.5 kgs. on 8th September, 1997. And my cholesterol level was down to 175.4 mg.

W.M. Bandusena
Sri Lanka

I am an angina patient since July, 1995. Second angiography in July, 1998 showed a marked deterioration of the blockages. I was advised angioplasty and I deposited advance money at Nanawati Hospital, Mumbai. On 18th July, I heard Dr. Chhajer's lecture at SNDT University and was so convinced that I took my money back from the hospital and decided to join his course in Delhi. I attended his course in August, 1998 and today I have come to attend the heart club. I can say that I am 75% cured. Initially my weight was 109 kgs. and after joining SAAOL my weight has come down to 102.6 kgs. I have lost more than 6 kgs. during the past 2 months. I used to take 5-6 tablets of sorbitrate but I have not taken any sorbitrate since August, 1998. Surprisingly I climbed the fifth floor of IMA, Delhi, where I stay (because the lift was out of order). I was very apprehensive in the beginning but when I started climbing, I went nonstop without any angina or dyspnea. This is really a miracle in two months. Yesterday I became confident and I am sure that my TMT will become negative in the next 6 months. My lipid profile has drastically improved and my angina has also disappeared. I am very grateful to him and his assistants who have given me a new and energetic life.

Dr. V.J.P. Sinha
Physician, Ghazipur, U.P.

On 8th May, 1997 at 2:30 a.m., I had a very severe pain in the chest and left shoulder. I was admitted to the local hospital and the doctor who attended my case confirmed that I had a heart attack. Due to lack of facilities I was shifted to Apollo Hospital and underwent an angiogram. There it was confirmed that I had three blockages each of 90%. Fortunately, I came to know through my relative about the SAAOL Heart Centre. From June 22nd-24th, 1997, I attended the program at Taj

Coramandal, Chennai. After a careful study of my heart problems, Dr. Bimal Chhajer advised me to strictly follow all that was imparted to me at SAAOL Heart Program. On my part, I started following the instructions right from the first day. I underwent a few regular tests to assess the improvements. I am extremely happy to present the following results:

Condition before joining SAAOL	Condition after 1 yr of joining SAAOL
Confirmed heart attack on 8.5.97. Blood pressure 200/110 mmHg	Average blood pressure 130/90mmHg
TMT positive as per test in June '97	TMT negative as per test in July '98
Recommended angioplasty/ bypass surgery	Zero oil diet, H.R.E., yoga meditation and Stress management
Drugs taken from May, 97 Betaloc-50mg, Ismo-250 mg Ecosprin-150mg, Ticlovas-250mg	Left drugs one by one Now I am only taking Ecosprin — one tablet after lunch
Weight as on 8.5.97/73kgs.	Weight as on 30.9.98/69kgs.
Serum lipid profile	Serum lipid profile
Total cholesterol 205 mg/dl HDL - 48 mg/dl LDL - 100 mg/dl Triglycerides - 162 mg/dl	Total cholesterol 180mg/dl HDL - 45 mg/dl LDL - 89 mg/dl Triglycerides - 140 mg/dl
I could only walk $^1/_2$ km. in 20 minutes	I walk every day at least for an hour. I also walked 14 km. at a stretch one day (Sabarimalai Temple)

Now I am proud to say, I am doing very well after joining the SAAOL Heart Program. My personal impressions are: i) I gained more self-confidence; ii) fully educated about the heart and its problems; iii) learnt more about food habits and zero oil diet. Thank you for the invitation on the occasion of 3rd anniversary celebrations which were held in New Delhi on 16th October, 1998. My family and friends join me in wishing the 3rd anniversary function of SAAOL every success.

V. Subramanian
Tamil Nadu

My mother joined the SAAOL (4th-7th, January 97) course in Badhkal. She is continuing to live actively and peacefully without any further complications; even at this advanced age of about 84 years, as a result of your training on improved life-style. She even does the HRE — health rejuvenating exercises daily, which you taught us and is living a totally independent life. I am grateful to you. She could not walk or work independently before joining your course because of angina pain. She sends you her blessings and good wishes. I too join her in that.

Jagdeshwari Devi's Son
A.K. Acharya, Govt. PG College
Hamirpur (H.P.)

On mid-noon of Feb. '98 I had to rush down to a client's office for some urgent work. Suddenly I felt some pain in the left upper corner of my chest which radiated to my left arm. It stopped on slowing down. I thought it must be some muscular pain, I need some regular exercise. The very next morning, I started my morning walk, but I felt the same pain just within 2-3 minutes of walking. Even after 4/5 days of morning walk the pain persisted. I knew I needed a doctor's help. He said it must be angina and I should have a TMT done. My TMT was highly positive and indicative of IHD.

My family physician referred me to a cardiologist. He advised me to get an angio done. With lots of mental preparation I went for my angio in April, 98, 70% obstruction in proximal lad — what next? My cardiologist advised me to have a thallium scan done to study the myocardial perfusion. Thallium scan re-confirmed "anteroseptal ischaema".

My bad days were on. I was told "lad supplies about 60% of the total supply to the heart walls and if I have an attack, it would be a fatal one and unmanageable," hence I should get an angioplasty done immediately. All my normal work was stopped, even the morning walk was not allowed.

I was declared hypertensive in 1998 and I took medicines for that. Then a few more were added:

(1) Tenormin LS one tablet, (2) Nicardia Retard 20 1BD, (3) Monotrate 10 1BD, (4) Ecospirin 150 one tab, (5) Ticlop 1BD, (6) Lopid 300 1BD, (7) Trika 0.5 after dinner.

No vitamins were added and the diet: normal except red meat and 1-2 eggs a week were allowed.

With this I started my financial planning as my medical insurance was not sufficient to cover such an expenditure. I requested my cardiologist to give me about three months before I go for angioplasty and stenting. I ran a small engineering manufacturing business and I needed some time to plan out things so that they did not go haywire in my absence. But I was refused any time. I consulted some more cardiologists in the town which led to even more confusion. Some advised "Immediate CABG". I was in deep trouble. I booked for "angioplasty and stenting", to be done by the best surgeon in Kolkata, on 27th May, 98. But one doctor friend of mine advised me not to get it done in Kolkata as my level of obstruction was very critical. Hence I booked my angioplasty in Chennai on 10th June, 98. I did not know what to do. My younger brother is a doctor in England. So I thought I would rather go to him. Also my *Mama*, maternal uncle, is a very senior neurologist in Mumbai, so I thought why not go to him. I really did not know what to do? A very famous cardio-thoracic surgeon from Mumbai comes to Kolkata once a week. I went to him with my angio film for his opinion. Frightening — he suggested an immediate CABG and he said within 6 months the obstruction will be 100% and I will not get any lasting relief by angioplasty. Hence I had no alternative but to go for CABG. That meant a lot of money for buying 10-12 years of extended life. I was only 48 years old, would 10-12 years be sufficient for me. My youngest daughter is 1985 born — that meant I would need a second CABG. I did my calculations and I felt so helpless that my engineering was of no help.

I made a copy of my angio film and sent it to my brother in England. The doctors there were also of the opinion that I should not go in for angioplasty but have a CABG done. So I started my financial planning and went for one final opinion to a very famous cardiologist, to know if I could wait till December so that I had sufficient time to organise things as I would be out of circulation for about 3 months if I went for a CABG. But he too suggested an immediate intervention, because in case in the meantime I had an attack, it would be very difficult to manage. Can you imagine my mental condition at that point of time? Then I sent another copy of the angio film to my *Mama* in Mumbai. They also suggested that angioplasty should not be tried at the proximal level — close to heart — rather I should try some cholesterol lowering drug and mild exercise to see if there is some improvement for the time being.

Suddenly my friend Somenath called my wife and told her about some doctor from Delhi suggesting an alternative to CABG about which he read in *The Statesman*.

Immediately I bought the newspaper and attended the free lecture by Dr. Bimal Chhajer. I found he was talking some sense. But it was really a very critical and tough decision to be taken at that moment. Somehow I gathered courage and decided to join the camp from 15th May, 98, considering that my hard-earned money (Rs. 12,000/- as course fee) might be a total loss. But I tell you, on completion of the camp, I was totally a different person, so confident, that nothing would happen to me. I cancelled all my hospital bookings and started the SAAOL program.

Under SAAOL program I again started my normal life and morning walk, HRE, yoga, stress management practices. I could not believe myself that within 15-20 days I started feeling much better. My lipids improved within 30 days. Gradually I increased my morning walk time and speed. Within 3 months I was walking about 5-6 kms in one hour. After 3 months I went for a TMT, really it was amazing. Although still positive there was a marked improvement. In August, I went with the reports to Dr. Chhajer and he was quite confident that within another 3 months time my TMT would be negative. In the meantime another *remarkable* thing had happened, my B.P. fell below normal and Dr. Chhajer advised me to withdraw Tenormin LS and Nicardia Retard. Can you believe, since 1998 I was maintaining my B.P. at 140/90 with the help of medicines and now I didn't require any medicines and my B.P. was 125/85. Is it not *startling*? Anyway I continued with my SAAOL program and now I walk about 7-8 kms in an hour and you know I am one of the fastest walkers in the Lakes and what more, no discomfort whatsoever. I'm so happy a person with all smiles. And do you know my present Lipids, total cholesterol is 120, triglycerides is 116 and the ratio of cholesterol : HDL is 4. Is it not really *astonishing*?

In November, I again went for TMT, oh no ! I just can't believe — it was Negative. I had got a new lease of life. It's really extraordinary. Dr. Chhajer is like GOD to me — I don't have words to thank him. He is beyond all these small thanks giving. He is great. He is too good. He is really working for an admirable cause.

Now I'm in Delhi. I have come here to get the thallium scan done at the Escorts. Today I went for my morning walk — from Safdarjung Enclave I walked down to the flyover near the Flying Club in 30 minutes. Tomorrow is my test. If that goes satisfactorily what word will I use to express my feelings — Astonishing! Amazing! Startling! or Miracle!

Rajani Mukherji on 11th December, 1998

It is really a miracle ! Dr. R.R. Kasliwal of Escorts commented: "It is a brilliant example — how much one can achieve by a proper life-style." My thallium scan is 100% normal — I am a normal person again — a new life.

I know, I don't have words to express my feelings. Still I would like to say, "Thanks" to Dr. Bimal Chhajer — "Thanks, Thanks, Thanks."

Rajani Mukherji
Kolkata - 700019

A GOAL

When the world looks gray
I was depressed and lost away
As MI made me down
Seemed that life was blown

Soon I found a way out
When life was trying to be knocked out
I found a goal
It was nothing but "SAAOL".

It's a wonderful family
To keep everyone hale and hearty
You feel enlightened from heart and soul
Once you come under the shelter of "SAAOL".

To keep you always out of depression
Just adopt everyday yoga and meditation
Diet and exercises are also the key
Excellent for everyone whether he or she.

At last health gets rejuvenated
Every movement gets fascinated
Let's make our one goal
Let everyone know it's only "SAAOL".

Jagdish Saran
New Delhi

I had a positive TMT in February, 1996 and underwent angioplasty with stent implantation, in February, 1996. Despite following the doctor's advice, I developed restenosis by July, 1996 and underwent another angioplasty in September, 1996.

I learnt from the *Economic Times* about SAAOL Program and attended a camp in January, 1997. I have been following the SAAOL program meticulously and my TMTs have been negative. I visited the Vaishno Devi shrine three days back. I climbed up and down without any discomfort. In fact this effort was very normal and pleasant.

V.K. Sood
Udaipur

It was on 7th January, 1998 that through one of my friends I came to know about "SAAOL", Dr. Bimal Chhajer and the program on "Reversal of Blockages". Meeting with Dr. Chhajer gave me hope and I decided to postpone the surgery and joined the program from 24th Jan. to 27th Jan. '98.

During the program I came to know that I had all the positive factors contributing to heart disease viz. obesity, smoking, lack of exercise, anger, high blood pressure, high cholesterol etc.

Now after about 5 months of attending the program and following it vigorously I have found a total change in my lifestyle. I have reduced my weight by 15 kgs. I only consume SAAOL tea twice a day. With the changing of life-style and following the SAAOL Heart Program strictly my TMT which was positive in Dec. '97 became negative in June, 98. This is all because of Dr. Chhajer and I thank him for the same, and advise others with similar problems to join the program and take benefits.

S.K. Bhatia

I had a heart attack in 1981 at the age of 38. It was a nightmare and I was mentally devastated. I used to play squash and tennis regularly. I had done regular exercise during my 16 years in the army. Though I was a bit overweight and smoked, yet it was difficult to believe that it could happen to me.

After my heart attack I went to USA to consult a leading heart institute. I followed the advice of cardiologists and gave up smoking and brought my weight down. I started exercising regularly but in 1986 I was back with heart problem and went again to USA where I underwent bypass surgery. I thought my problems were over and I exercised regularly, controlled my weight and cholesterol. Despite all precautions, I was back in USA in 1990 with problems of chest pain. I underwent bypass surgery once again. I controlled all the factors that could aggravate my heart disease after the surgery. Despite that, my TMT last done in May, 1998 was positive. Nightmare of a third bypass surgery again started to haunt me. I knew I had to look for an alternative.

Though I had heard of SAAOL Heart Program way back in 1995 and had read Dr. Dean Ornish's book in 1990, yet I was a sceptical. I could not believe that someone could be so different from all the surgeons and cardiologists who had been working in some of the best hospitals in the world. How could someone be so radically different and yet have a simple approach to heart disease.

I joined the SAAOL Program thinking, "There is nothing wrong if someone has a different approach." Well I have finished the program. For me, who has lived with this problem for 17 years, it has been an eye opener. This is the first time I have felt confident that I stand a better chance of reversing my disease. I only wish SAAOL had given more information in their advertisements to attract my attention many years ago. I would recommend this program to all those who have the disease and for all those who may get heart disease.

S.P. Khosla
Businessman, Delhi

In 1988 I had a heart attack. In 1989, Dr. Kaul in AIIMS performed my PTCA which failed. So immediately, I went for bypass surgery by Dr. Venugopal. The problem recurred after a few years and I feared a repeat of angina. Gradually, the condition became so bad that I could barely walk 10-15 steps. During this time I discovered that my blood sugar (fasting - 108 mg%), total cholesterol (292.5 mg%) and triglycerides (223.9 mg%) were all quite high. I was advised an angiogram. Knowing the consequences of angiogram well, I decided to join SAAOL.

I joined the course immediately on 5th September, 1998. I followed everything especially diet and medications strictly and religiously. Now after 5½ months of joining, my report of blood sugar (Fasting - 69 mg%), total cholesterol (136.7 mg%) of triglycerides (126 mg%) have all come down drastically to my satisfaction. Moreover, I can now walk continuously for ½ an hour without any breathlessness or discomfort. I attend all parties and social gatherings and have never felt that I was missing anything.

Getting a bypass surgery done is not all that a patient needs. Unless he changes his life-style, the problem comes back. I would advise all the people to follow SAAOL before considering a bypass (or repeat bypass). I would like to thank SAAOL Heart Program as I am normal again and half of my angina medicines have been withdrawn in the last 5½ months.

Thanks to SAAOL for this improvement in me.

Shiv Narain Malhotra
Businessman, New Delhi.

I joined the course in August 1997, after having second M.I. in June '97. My first M.I. was in February '91 and then bypass was done in the same year. After joining and following the SAAOL treatment, I am living a comfortable life now. I do yoga, walking and meditation everyday and am also doing the zero oil treatment. Now I don't feel any chest pain or breathlessness.

In December, 1997 a complete check-up was done and found TMT negative, cholesterol level had also come down.

Ramesh Kumar Arora
New Delhi

In March, 1998 when I was to go abroad I had undergone tests for medical inspection when the ECG showed some abnormality. So TMT was taken on 24/3/98 (at Mumbai) which was positive.

On my return in July, 1998 I attended Dr. Chhajer's talk and joined the camp in IMC, Mumbai from 30/8/98 to 1/9/98. Thereafter I religiously followed the food regimen, advocated HRE, yoga and meditation, except when I used to go out of Mumbai.

After 7 months of the SAAOL observation I took TMT on 19/3/99 at Mumbai Hospital. The report was negative. As regards cholesterol it has improved from 197 mg/dl in Aug, 1998 to 173 mg/dl on 18/3/99.

I can walk long distances now without getting tired. I must confess that as regards yoga and meditation I haven't been able to adhere to the strict observance due to paucity of time though in HRE I am regular.

My aim is to discard the medicines which have been prescribed to me and I am assured that with the improvement that I have made till now, I should be in a position to achieve my objective.

G.B. Bhooshanan
Retd. Jt. Chief Officer, RBI

I had an MI on 12/8/98. Angioplasty was done on 22/8/98 for RCA which was 99% blocked on angiography. It also showed 80% block on LAD for which the doctor advised another angioplasty. In the meantime I came across Dr. Chhajer's program which I attended on 4th June, 1999.

Friends, after attending Dr. Chhajer's program for 3 days and following his directions regarding food, meditation, exercise, Kayotsarga my quality of life has improved. My TMT is negative. I feel inspired and fit in just 3 months.

Regarding zero-oil diet my wife, daughter and I get together and make a planned menu for one full week from various choices. I get pleasure waiting for certain items on a particular day and my wife enjoys preparing it. This, I think, adds value to our eating ...

Dr. D. Hurbada
Medical Practitioner, Mumbai

Being a follower of SAAOL Heart Program, let me thank you at the outset for having come to the rescue of several thousands of CHD patients.

Let me narrate my experience with SAAOL Heart Program. I had a heart attack in 1990. When an angiography was taken, I had 5 blocks, 1st of 100%, 2nd of 75% and 3rd below 75%. I was recommended bypass surgery. Since I had some financial difficulties to meet the bypass surgery cost, I took a second medical opinion. Then I was told to continue with my medication and low-salt and low-fat food. I had continued this and there was no problem. When I retired from my service in 1996, I started taking my normal food without any restriction on oil as I was under the impression that my blocks had dissolved. However, in January 1998, I again had a problem of angina. Again I underwent an angiography, it was reported that I had blocks, 1st of 100%, 2nd of 90%, 3rd of 80%, 4th of 75%. I was recommended immediate bypass surgery. I had fixed my surgery for 14/4/1998. I had read in one of the old newspapers about SAAOL Heart Program conducted by Dr. Bimal Chhajer in January, 1998. Immediately I contacted Mr. Deepak Dalal, Program Coordinator of Dr. Bimal Chhajer in Mumbai and bought the booklet published by them. I followed the guidance given therein. Within a week I could feel some improvement in my angina problem. So I attended his camp at Lonavala in April, 1998. As my angiography was taken in February, 1998, I was to undergo a bypass within 3 months, i.e. by May, 1998. So I underwent a blood test which showed a marked improvement in my cholesterol and triglycerides level. This gave me encouragement and I cancelled my bypass surgery appointment. There was no looking back since I attended the SAAOL Camp. Given below are my blood test reports conducted periodically every 3 months since March, 1998. I have also undergone TMT twice which has also become negative. I am now waiting for a non-invasive angiography to ascertain how far my blocks have reduced. Just imagine, my waist was 40 inches in March, 1998. Now it is 33 inches. My weight and other details are given below:

As my CHD was in an advanced stage, my family members were very worried and they insisted that I should undergo bypass surgery immediate-ly. When I was in the SAAOL Camp, my wife who had accompanied me was so worried and was under the impression that I was avoiding bypass surgery and there was an imminent likelihood of a fatal heart attack. She left the camp half-way. Now they are all convinced about SAAOL Heart Program and my wife is cooking my food without a drop of oil.

We are all grateful and indebted to Dr. Bimal Chhajer for this excellent line of medical management for CHD patients.

N.S. Hariharan
Service Person, Mumbai

On 12/5/99 I had undergone the TMT test. It was negative. The doctor told me "You are not a heart patient at all. Which doctor asked you to take medicines for heart disease." I said, "Doctor six months back my TMT was positive." The doctor was surprised again and asked the doctor's name who had performed the TMT test. He couldn't believe that a positive TMT could become negative. I said it was a long story. I will explain it all to you some other time.

The following is the story of my positive TMT changing to negative TMT which was unbelievable to the doctors in Roorkee.

I am 38 years old, had angina pain last year. As the TMT was positive doctors in Apollo Hospital, Chennai advised me angiography and angioplasty. But after attending Dr. Chhajer's camp in Chennai in Octo-ber, 1998, I started following all the instructions advised by SAAOL doc-tors. I changed my life-style and I have made a tremendous achieve-ment after only six months. There is no angina pain. My TMT which was positive (6 mins) is now negative. I am thankful to God and have no words to thank Dr. Chhajer. May SAAOL continue to lead in helping the suffering people having heart problems.

N.H. Ansari
Roorkee

Iam G. Karmakar from West Bengal, staying at Dilshad Garden, Delhi. It is my privilege to talk to you about SAAOL. My son-in-law Shri Anup K. Chakraborty enrolled me for the SAAOL camp.

Since last year I had little pain in my chest. When the pain kept recur-ring for a long time my family doctor advised me to go for an angiogra-phy. I had my angiography done from Ram Manohar Lohia Hospital. The results showed that the arteries were 60% and 80% blocked. The doctor advised me to undergo bypass surgery at the earliest.

I joined the SAAOL program on the 2nd of April, 1999 with my wife. We derived immense pleasure and satisfaction, particularly on the last day when personal attention was given by the doctors, specially Dr. Chhajer who spoke to me in Bengali. The excellent part of this training was when he gave examples from day-to-day life and expressed his viewpoint clearly, for example on stress.

I no longer feel any angina pain in my chest. Previous medication could not give me the relief that I feel at present after following the SAAOL Program. On 2nd April, 1999 my weight was 75 kgs. After taking all the advice given by SAAOL, my weight has reduced by 5 kgs. in one month.

I am taking an oil free diet, doing yoga, exercises, doing morning walk etc. as directed by Dr. Chhajer. This has not only made me healthy, but I am also living more satisfied and fuller life.

Thank God that I joined this program and am very grateful to Dr. Bimal Chhajer.

G. Karmakar
Delhi

Modern life-style in reality is a death style

The biggest killer in the world today accounting for almost 80% deaths worldwide is not war, disease, natural calamities or accidents, but life-style! Now what is this modern life-style? Who are its major culprits? How do they manifest unknowingly in our body? Read the following and THINK!

"What is this life, if full of styles

Which slow poison your mind and body futile

Natural healthy styles out, deadly artificial styles in

Comforts, conveniences, pollutions and junk foods galore

Physical, mental, spiritual exercises nil.

Increasing obesity, stress, sugar, salt and oil

Breeding silent killers: cholesterol, diabetes, aids and cancer causes

Producing heart disease, depression and psychic disorders

No time for own family, elders and self but

Plenty for late nights, smoke, drinks, harmful foods.

No mood to love and no concern for kin.

Constantly in mad race for money and win

At any cost and by any and all means.

As survival of fittest the only thumb rule.

Or else, odd man out, and you a silly fool.

Enough money for false esteem and show off

Falling prey to unscrupulous elements

No time for long-term relationships and priorities.

Plenty for short-term options and gains

Finally it's too late at crossroads of death

Hence healthy food for thought and eye-opener.

I had my money and my health.

I strained my health to get more wealth.

I spent my wealth to regain health.

I lost my health and my wealth."

Narendra N. Shethia
Mumbai

On January, 1998 I got a massive heart attack and was admitted to Apollo, Chennai. For three days I was in ICU and for a week more in the hospital. Then I was advised 3 months of bed rest with simple diet and regular medicines. I was advised immediate angiography.

There were divergent views about angiography. My fear was that it leads to the operation theatre. At this critical juncture a blessing in disguise came through Dr. Chhajer's lecture which I attended. To my happiness, the lecture educated me that the angiography apart from being superfluous is injurious too. Immediately I decided to attend the camp with my wife in May 1998.

The three-day camp changed our entire life-style. The medication, meditation, exercise, walking and "0" oil diet with cooking demonstration brought new life to me.

I have strictly adhered to the SAAOL system and periodically attended all the camps subsequently and brought my weight down to the proper level together with cholesterol HDL, B.P., Echo, etc.

Exactly after one year in the month of May, 1999 my TMT was found negative. The entire credit goes to SAAOL Heart Program and Dr. Chhajer.

I would like to mention here that every aspect of the programme has a bearing on our life and our actions, small or big.

Gobind Singh Bajaj
Chennai

I was suffering from heart disease since last year. I am diabetic also for the last 10-11 years, taking all the prescribed medicines regularly. On 11th January, 1999, I was advised to go for angiography and angioplasty by my cardiologist as I was having pain in the chest since November, 1998. I had seen the ad in the newspaper by Dr. Bimal Chhajer MD, recommending REVERSAL OF HEART DISEASE with new doctrine and change of life-style, diet and yoga exercise, meditation and discarding angioplasty and bypass surgery. I therefore visited him on 01/02/99 and joined the camp from 05 to 07 February, 1999.

The 1st day, when I attended the camp, I was unable to sit on a chair for half an hour due to pain and discomfort in the chest. Thus I had to sit on a mat on the floor, arrangement for which was already there. During the camp and thereafter, till today, I had not met even a single man who attended his camp and said that he had not benefited from this treatment. That encouraged me a lot.

My pain vanished in almost 2 weeks after starting his full follow up with medicines. During the camp, they actually teach the patient to be at least half a doctor about this trouble. At present I am much above average in this short time. My blood cholesterol decreased with the diet change of zero oil food and with rest of the follow-up as below:

02/02/99   31/03/99   09/06/99

(249.00 mgs/dl)   (160.00 mgs/dl)   (150.00 mgs/dl)

By eating zero oil food with fibre, my blood sugar also went down a great deal from 204 (fasting) on 14/09/98 to 142.00 (fasting) on 09/06/99 without any change in medicines. I may add here that all my family members enjoyed zero oil vegetarian. lunch since the day I started this program. As I have the experience now, I am sure that heart disease cannot be stopped with medicines only, unless one changes the one's life-style, zero oil diet and that too vegetarian only, rejuvenating exercises, asanas and management of stress. This is a type of health insurance without any payment in cash, though you should not discard the medicines without the advice of your cardiologist and SAAOL, the rehabilitation experts. I wish Dr. Chhajer, MD a long life to promote this program for years to come. May God bless him.

T.R. Chadha
New Delhi

On 10th January, 1993 I had a heart attack and subsequently had cerebral thrombosis (stroke) with left side paralysis on 1st December, 1994. Paralysis persisted for two days with blood sugar f (106), cholesterol (385), triglycerides (191), LDL (315) and HDL (32). The problems of angina recurred after a few years and my health deteriorated. Gradually the condition became so bad that I could barely walk 10-15 steps and I was advised angiography. Accordingly I was ready to proceed to Escorts Hospital, Delhi for angiography and bypass surgery. But with the strong recommendation of my sister, I joined the SAAOL Heart Program on 27th November, 1998 at Kolkata. The course changed my life completely and now I can not only walk continuously for ½ an hour without any problem but can regularly jog for 5 minutes with improving reports of cholesterol (175), triglycerides (141), Blood Sugar (83)F.

If anybody wants to get rid of heart disease permanently, join Dr. Bimal Chhajer's SAAOL Heart Program immediately.

Soumen Bose
Durgapur

I am a diabetic. I generally have an annual medical check-up. In last year's medical check-up, my stress test was positive. I consulted a cardiac surgeon. He suggested that I should get an echocardiogram and stress thallium scan. The echo was normal and the thallium scan was positive. Therefore, they suggested I should have an angiogram done. I was surprised since my other health parameters were normal. Fortunately, I had no symptoms. Therefore, I decided to wait.

Meanwhile, there was a write up about Dr. Bimal K. Chhajer's SAAOL Heart Program scheduled in Bangalore. My wife and myself attended the course which was very impressive.

So, I started zero oil vegetarian diet, meditation, yoga and half an hour's walk daily or played golf for the last seven months.

In order to monitor the progress, I had a check-up. My diabetic parameters had come down below normal. My doctor reduced the medicines to half. The thallium scan indicated good exercise tolerance. Dr. Chhajer who saw the test reports said that the blood flow to the heart is more and my stress test was negative. I certainly consider it as good progress. I feel more confident, less stressful with improvement in my health.

I congratulate Dr. Chhajer and his colleagues for following the unchartered path, unlike the present technologically driven route of angiography, angioplasty and bypass surgery.

A.A. Raju
Industrial Management Consultant

I had two heart attacks, one was in 1976 and the other was in 1994,viz., eighteen years later. I have diabetes mellitus for the past six years.

On 29/5/98, I experienced pain in the centre of my chest and then it radiated towards the right. I consulted my cardiologist. He suggested I undergo an angiography test. On enquiry, I was told by him that this was a complicated test and one out of 1500 patients who undergo it dies. This is a common test to know the blockages in coronary arteries. I was extremely scared and desperate. I did not know how to proceed in the matter. I consulted two more cardiologists in Bangalore. They also suggested coronary angiography.

My wife somehow was reluctant and I obliged her by not undergoing this test. One fine day, I received a call from my wife's sister that one Dr. Bimal Chhajer is delivering a lecture on "Reversing heart disease". She asked us to attend the lecture. We heard his lecture for nearly 2 hours with rapt attention. This was in June, 1998. On the same day we decided to join Bimal Chhajer's SAAOL Program from 29/6/98 to 1/7/98.

According to my previous "Two dimensional-colour doppler studies — echocardiogram report" I was diagnosed to have "hypertrophic cardiomyopathy". After going through the report, Dr. Chhajer was of the strong opinion that I was not a patient of cardiomyopathy and angiography was as prescribed by previous cardiologist was not necessary in view of my heart efficiency being 63 per cent. From the SAAOL program, I could understand that this was a tremendous opportunity to lead a more meaningful, balanced and full life. I followed the zero oil diet, meditation, medication and exercise taught in the course fully, for the last one year which has yielded remarkable results. *During September, 98 I underwent TMT as suggested by Dr. Chajjer which to our surprise was found to be negative.* My weight has reduced considerably by 6 to 7 kgs. in a period of 4 months and I maintained this weight throughout. There is a considerable reduction in blood sugar and cholesterol levels. My glycosylated haemoglobin is less than seven. Here is the table:

	Before SAAOL Treatment	One Year after SAAOL treatment
Fasting blood sugar	101	75
Post prandial sugar	160	145
Serum cholesterol	236	151
Serum triglycerides	156	141
HDL	32.7	33.9
LDL	119.9	88
TMT	Positive	Negative

I have not experienced any chest pain afterwards. Change in life-style has made me very comfortable. I can talk about my heart, feeling better than before. Whenever I come in contact with heart patients, I talk about my experience of heart disease and change of life-style taught by Dr. Chhajer. This course is very educative. I can communicate better to speak from the heart instead of only from the head.

G.V. Raman
Bangalore

What newspapers say about us

More than 200 news articles and reports have been published on the SAAOL Heart Program in the last few years. A few of the titles are reproduced here. In addition, the SAAOL Heart Program has been covered in the news on DD2 (Aaj Tak), ANI, DD1, etc.

1. An Open Heart Story — how to look after your heart — *Life Positive*, October, 1996

2. Bypassing Surgery — *India Today*, April 15, 1996

3. Bypassing Surgery — *The Week*, February 18, 1996

4. Bypassing the Bypass — *The Indian Express* (All Editions), December 17, 1997

5. SAAOL Beat: The SAAOL Heart Program tackles heart trouble with diet and exercise — *Mid-day*, Mumbai, October 15, 1997

6. Bypass and Angioplasty surgeries can be avoided — *Express Newsline*, New Delhi, September 29, 1997

7. Most Bypass Surgeries avoidable — *Deccan Herald*, Bangalore, September 28, 1997

8. Cardiologist prescribes drug free cure — *Newsline*, Chandigarh, August 1, 1997

9. Take care of your heart — *The Times of India*, New Delhi, June 17, 1997

10. Simple lifestyle can reduce Heart Disease — *The Hindustan Times*, New Delhi, June 12, 1997

11. Simple lifestyle can reverse Heart Blockages — *The Asian Age*, June 12, 1997

12. An Interview with Dr. Chhajer - "From the Doctor's Desk" — *The Telegraph*, Kolkata, May 26, 1997

13. Bypassing the Bypass — *The Hindu*, Business Line, May 6, 1997 (All Editions)

14. Himalayan Task — *Kalki* (Tamil Magazine), Chennai, May 4, 1997

15. Mayor inaugurates SAAOL Heart Program — *News Today*, Chennai, April 26, 1997

16. Cheering hearts — *Outlook*, January 26, 1998

17. Matters of the heart — *Life Positive*, October, 1998

18. A new technique to reverse heart blockages — *The Hindustan Times*, October 5, 1998

19. Cardiologist's prescription slip has a new word — yoga — *Express Newsline*, November 28, 1999

20. Disciplined life key to good health— *The Asian Age*, November 28, 1999

21. Heart ailments caused by lifestyle — *The Statesman*, November 24, 1999

22. Know your coronary risk score — *The Times of India*, November 24, 1999

23. Change lifestyle to avoid heart attack — *The Hindustan Times*, November 24, 1999

24. Prescription for the new millennium — *Financial Express*, November 21, 1999
25. Getting into the heart of your lifestyle — *The Times of India,* November 17, 1999
26. Reversal of heart blockage is possible — *Medivision*, November 1-5, 1999

My views about other therapies

Today so many alternative therapies exist which claim to help in controlling heart disease. Reiki, Hydrotherapy, Garlic Therapy, Massage, Meditation and Pranic Healing are few of them. A lot of people ask me whether they can wear a magnet, copper band, rudraksh chain in the neck and so on. The only advice I give them is: "do whatever does not interfere with the SAAOL System — if it helps to cut down your worries it will definitely be of help." Even a belief in God or the blessings of a Guru help. Go for anything that does not contain oil or excess fat or cholesterol.

Homeopathy, Ayurveda, Unani etc. can also be of help in heart disease — but I am not an expert in these fields. If you have diabetes — ask your homeopath to avoid sweet tablets. Do not consume any ghee or oil which is often mixed in many Ayurveda preparations. In fact, I also recommend a special herbal tea — the SAAOL tea for treating heart disease.

Medical science discovers new items every day — may be they will find natural herbs useful in heart care. Till the research is completed and proofs are available medical science may not recommend them but I do not object if is there no harm. But do follow the life-style that I recommend.

Some other heart diseases

Other Presentations of heart disease

Though coronary heart disease is the most common of all heart diseases, there are still a variety of other diseases which affect the heart, causing morbidity and a significant reduction in the efficiency of the functions of the heart.

1. Congenital heart disease

For the perfect functioning of the heart, a normal and healthy heart with normal valves and muscular walls is necessary. Some children are born with defective valves or defective partitions between the walls which separate different chambers of the heart. This is known as congenital heart disease.

Many of these defects, which are insignificant, generally get healed by themselves or do not cause any discomfort and handicap throughout one's lifetime. But if the defect is major, it ultimately requires correction or replacement by surgery.

2. Rheumatic heart disease

This is one of the common causes of defect in the valves of the heart. It mostly occurs in childhood but the manifestations may come even later in life. Breathlessness and enlargement of the heart are the main complaints.

The cause of the disease is an auto-immune response of the body following a throat infection. Rheumatic heart disease in children and young adults must be treated with a monthly injection of penicillin till 25 years of age. Many patients may ultimately need surgery.

3. Cardiomyopathy

In this disease there is a gradual weakening of heart muscles and the heart gradually enlarges. Most of the cases are due to myocardial ischaemia (deficiency of blood and oxygen) or coronary heart disease. Many infections also predispose to cardiomyopathy, specially viral infections.

4. Diseases of irregular heartbeats (Cardiac Arrhythmias)

In a wide variety of such diseases the heartbeat or the rhythm of the heart becomes abnormal. There are irregular beats and the rate is reduced (brady arrhythmia) or increased (tachy arrhythmia). The either patient may complain of unconsciousness, palpitations or missing the beats. These diseases are due to the damage in the pacemaker or the conduction system of the heart. Majority of these problems aggravate with mental stress and are due to lack of blood supply and oxygen (due to coronary artery blockages). Drugs and temporary pacemaker implantations are temporary treatments, but a life-style change and stress reduction can lead to a permanent relief from these diseases.

SAAOL Health and Research Foundation (SHARF)

This charitable society has recently been registered with the Medical Society in order to spread awareness about proper lifestyle, diet and stress management. I have started a new concept to reach the masses to make my dream of prevention and cure of heart disease a reality.

This is a very small organization. Only your help and support can promote this organization and make SAAOL a movement.

**The objectives and aims of SHARF
are as follows:**

1. To carry out research on reversal of coronary heart disease and lowering its risk factors.
2. To spread education in the science of health, yoga and meditation.
3. To continue supporting heart patients, who need to follow the SAAOL life-style.
4. To organize seminars, programs, functions and lectures by persons of high spiritual orders and the preachers of philosophy of "Non-violence", "*Preksha*", "*Jeevan Vigyan*" and "*Anekant*", and scholars of outstanding national and international fame.
5. To publish bulletins, journals, books, reports, research and work papers with a view to propagate knowledge on matters relevant to or falling within the purview of the objects of the Society.

Activities of the SAAOL heart club

SAAOL Heart Club

Clubs and organizations are in plenty where get-togethers take place. Since we were holding regular get-togethers for heart patients to we decided to hold such meetings under the banner of **SAAOL Heart Club.** This unique club only has members who have heart ailments or related risk factors — A *club exclusively for heart patients.*

The aim of the club is to continuously monitor and help our

participants. The club started and was inaugurated by the re-nowned doctor turned political activist Dr. J. K. Jain on 2nd March, 1996 at Suraj Kund Resort.

The club meetings are held once a month since it has been established. Medical examinations are carried out every time and SAAOL lunch is served to the members apart from revision training of yoga and meditation. Every meeting is focused on a special topic of discussion. Let me record the special focus of all the Heart Club meetings held so far :

2nd March, 1996: A talk by the famous cardiologist Dr. P. D. Nigam, Padmashree, former head of cardiology, Dr. Ram Manohar Lohia Hospital, New Delhi and a consultant cardiologist in Apollo Indraprastha Hospital, New Delhi.

7th April, 1996: A talk by Dr. Deepak Natrajan, a young cardiologist who is the head of the department of cardiology in Dr. Ram Manohar Lohia Hospital, New Delhi. He spoke on Preventive Cardiology. Dr. Natrajan was all praise for whatever we were doing.

5th May, 1996: A talk by Dr. Rakesh Verma. MD, DM. Dr. Verma is heading the department of cardiology in Safdarjung Hospital, one of the oldest hospitals in Delhi. Dr. Verma appreciated the efforts put in by the club to increase the awareness of the members.

2nd June, 1996: Two guest speakers were there in this meeting.

Dr. Rahul Malhotra, a young cardiologist and director of the upcoming Malhotra Heart Institute, spoke on the trends of heart disease prevalence and treatment in India and USA. Dr. Malhotra praised the activities of SAAOL in India.

Prof. N. P. Singh — the executive director of Green Cross Society demonstrated cardiac resuscitation for the patients. He used models to show what to do in an emergency when someone is lying unconscious or has had a heart attack. The participants greatly appreciated the event.

7th July, 1996: The speaker of this meeting was Dr. S. Padmawati, the most famous name in the field of cardiology in India. She is the Chief of National Heart Institute in Delhi. She spoke on Preventive Cardiology. She was also our judge for the SAAOL Food Cooking Competition, and appreciated the varieties of oil-free food, which were served in the meeting.

20th July, 1996: SAAOL Heart Club/ SAAOL Health and Research Foundation organized a seminar on: Heart Care Awareness — The Role Of Media, in collaboration with the Indian Express Group. The list of speakers was very impressive:

Dr. Pratap C. Reddy, Chairman, Apollo group of hospitals.

Dr. J. K. Jain, Director, Jain Medical Center, New Delhi.

Prof. K. S. Reddy, Prof. Cardiology, All India Institute Of Medical Sciences, New Delhi.

Dr. K. L. Chopra, Chief, Heart Care Foundation, New Delhi.

Dr. Rahul Malhotra, Director, Malhotra Heart Institute, New Delhi.

Dr. Naresh Trehan, Chief, Escorts Heart Institute, New Delhi. (Dr. Trehan could not ultimately make it and was represented by his colleague Dr. Mehral)

Dr. Bimal Chhajer MD., Director of SAAOL Heart Program.

4th August, 1996: It was a SAAOL family picnic in a beautiful farmhouse owned by one of our members, Mr. A. L. Jain in Bijwasan, Delhi. It was a great change for the members who enjoyed the Quiz, Antakshari and Games.

1st October, 1996: Annual function of SAAOL Heart Club was celebrated. There was a cultural program followed by a dinner at the PHD Chamber of Commerce Hall.

2nd October, 1996: A complete one day revision course of

SAAOL Heart Program was held at Acharya Sushil Muni Ashram, Defence Colony. This one day course was attended by eighty members where they practised and recollected all that they had learnt during the SAAOL course. Many outstation patients also attended it.

3rd November, 1996: SAAOL Heart Quiz was organized at our favourite resort at Suraj Kund where the club members had to answer 40 questions on how heart diseases occur, what foods prevent heart diseases and so on. More than 100 people participated. The winners, Dr. R. K. Bhatnagar, Dr. Raghunath Airi and Mr. V. P. Kapoor were given attractive prizes.

8th December, 1996: Winter is the time for plenty of fruits and vegetables. We organized a Food Exhibition and Salad Making Competition at Badhkal Lake Resort. Hundreds of members visited the exhibition and learned the contents of different foods and their caloric values.

5th January, 1997: The new year of the club started with a Poster Exhibition on coronary heart disease. Our doctors, dieticians and colleagues prepared more than 75 posters on different aspects of heart disease. The SAAOL lunch was a special attraction.

2nd February, 1997: The focus of this meeting was a talk by Dr. Chhajer on "Physical Activity and Heart Disease". Heart patients were informed how to calculate physical activity and all relevant details. Queries were answered.

9th March, 1997: Stress and Heart Disease was the theme of the talk in this meeting and Type-A and Type-B Behaviours of people were explained. All the members assessed themselves for Type-A behaviour. Members were explained how heart disease is closely related to stress.

13th April, 1997: The focus of discussion was: Scientific Research on Yoga. More than hundred members attended.

4th May, 1997: We organized a Diet Quiz in this meeting.

This generated tremendous enthusiasm. Different food items were demonstrated and the fat and calorie contents were discussed.

8th June, 1997: Many of our participants wanted to know about High Blood Pressure. So Dr. Chhajer gave a talk on all the aspects of hypertension. Medical examination of all the members was carried out as usual. Meditation revision class was led by Shri B .L. Jain.

6th July, 1997: Heart Club discussion topic for this month was Diabetes Mellitus. Dr. Chhajer gave a detailed account of how diabetes develops and how it can predispose to heart disease.

10th August, 1997: The topic this week was Obesity or Overweight. Dr. Chhajer used beautiful transparencies to explain about different aspects of obesity in this meeting.

7th September, 1997: Many of our members were still confused about the lipids, so Dr. Chhajer delivered a detailed talk on Lipid Story. Triglycerides, HDL cholesterol, fatty acids, cholesterol, saturated, mono-unsaturated, polyunsaturated fat — all these terms were elaborated and explained in this meeting. Mr. L. K. Jha led the meditation session. Dr. Nehal Ahmad and Dr. Vishal Sharma carried out the medical examinations and follow-ups and Mr. Trehan demonstrated some yoga postures.

5th October, 1997: Importance of Meditation on Reversal of Heart Disease and Its Help in Reopening of Blockages in CHD. Topics covered : scientific and medical basis for which meditation is employed by SAAOL.

5th November, 1997: Investigations which confirm the Reversal of Blockages in the Coronary Blood Vessels. Topics covered : Changes which appear and indicate the presence of heart disease. How to assess improvement. Latest investigations as MRI Angio, PET Scan. Dr. Airi, our old participant, released his new book of Hindi poems.

7th December, 1997 : Food Exhibition and Cooking Competition
Theme : 'Dieticians — Doctors of tomorrow': a unique exhibition organised jointly by SHARF and Haryana Tourism Corporation. Topics covered : Selection of proper food. Increasing awareness of the scientific aspects of food and cooking. Foods commonly consumed along with their nutritive values, disease prevention capacity and conversion factors. Cooking competition.

4th January, 1998 : SAAOL Risk Scoring. More than 70 people participated and assessed their control and reversal potentials to the date.

25th January, 1998 : Health Food Festival Jointly organised by SAAOL and Haryana Tourism Corporation. Included Cooking Competition, Health Quiz and Baby Show.

8th March, 1998 : Fat Distribution in the Body and How to Lose Fat Important for those who are overweight.

12th April, 1998 : Overview of Number of Heart Patients in India, Approximate Number of Bypasses, Angioplasties Performed." Dr. Chhajer pointed out that most angioplasties and bypasses can be avoided if doctors and cardiologists advise proper lifestyle modifications.

3rd May, 1998 : Relation Between High Blood Pressure, Diabetes, Obesity and CHD. Dr. Chhajer pointed out that though this topic is generally discussed in medical conferences, he has simplified it to make facts more clear for people who are non-medicos.

7th June, 1998 : Role of Antioxidants. Topics covered : Vitamins A, C, E as Wonder Drugs/Magic Foods to help retard the blockages and reverse them. What are antioxidants? Sources, research studies, preparations available in the market. How much to consume?

12th July, 1998 : Physical Activity and Heart. Topics covered :

Kinds of exercises and yoga. What is best for the common man and heart disease in modern times.

2nd August, 1998 : Socio-behavioural and Environmental Factors in Heart Disease. Topics covered : Why Indians are more prone to heart disease? The cultural, economical, retirement factors. Ways to change them.

5th September, 1998 : Yoga in Heart Disease and Stress Relief. Lecture by learned yoga expert Swami D. Yogesh, founder and chairman of Vatika Yogashram, Delhi. He enlightened the participants on better aspects of yoga, and meditation. He also discussed how yoga and meditation together help to manage stress.

October 1998: How to Increase Weight for those who were underweight and what to do if the blood pressure is also low. We had a good gathering of our old participants and there was also a lunch after Dr. Chhajer's lecture.

November, 1998 : Story of Cholesterol. Dr. Chhajer discussed the structure and SAAOL values of cholesterol for prevention and reversal of blockages.

December, 1998 : Diseases related to stress *(Psychosomatic Diseases).* Since heart disease is very much stress related we thought of discussing some of the most important stress related diseases which occur simultaneously with the heart disease and have a common origin from stress.

January, 1999 : Guest lecture was given by Dr. Arvind Lal, Director of Dr. Lal's pathological lab and leading pathologist. He spoke about common tests like the lipid profile and blood glucose-fasting and post prandial and showed beautiful illustrations on slides.

February, 1999 : Pollution and its Effect on Health. Dr. Chhajer discussed the hazards of pollution which were causing a series of harmful diseases.

March, 1999 : Sweet making competition. At Holi, the festival of colours and sweets, we had a great variety of oil-free sweets made by our participants. Prizes were given to the best three.

April, 1999 : How our Personalities are Stress Related. Dr. Chhajer had permulated a personality score in which many of our participants took part.

May, 1999 : SAAOL Playing Cards. 52 tips for a healthy heart were discussed and presented in the form of playing cards.

June, 1999 : The topic discussed was *SAAOL Treatment of Bronchial Asthma.*

July, 1999 : Identification of Hostile People. Types of personalities were discussed and how to deal with hostile people.

August, 1999 : "How to assess your work stress and how to handle these stresses." A scoring was formulated.

12th September, 1999 : Sectors of life Self Analysis.

10th October 1999 : Competition of Zero Oil Snacks and Namkeens.

14th November 1999 : Namkeen Competition. A Namkeen cooking competition and an exhibition of namkeen was organized. A lot of enthusiasm was shown by the participants.

12th December 1999 : How to become successful in life?. Steps to a successful person and basic qualities of a successful personality were discussed.

16th January 2000 : Meditation and Stress Management Part-1. A detailed discussion on stress, its production and the common features of different kinds of meditation.

13th February 2000 : How to Measure Stress — from the Medical View? Stress is the most important risk factor for heart disease and other life-style diseases. A discussion on ways of diagnosing and measuring stress.

12th March 2000 : Alternative Medicine. A discussion on different kinds of existing alternative systems.

9th April 2000 : Constipation — A Common Problem for Heart Patients. A discussion on what constipation is, what are its causes and treatment. A classification of medicines which can be used for curing constipation was given.

14th May 2000 : Cholesterol, Triglycerides and the Liver. A discussion on structure, functions, absorption, production of cholesterol, common drugs, which can lower cholesterol-triglycerides and their mechanism of action.

11th June 2000 : Today's children due to bad life-style and stresses are prone to risk of developing coronary heart disease. A discussion on how to prevent it was carried out.

16th July 2000 : A Heart quiz was organized for participants.

13th August 2000 : Dr. Chhajer discussed about the *Executive Health Checkup.*

10th September 2000 : How to check the improved stress Management Skills? Special Stress Analysis Cards were distributed on that Day.

8th October 2000 : Aging is a gradual and continuous process and an inevitable change in every person's life. Dr. Chhajer delivered an informative and interesting talk on *How to Age Gracefully after 45 years of Age.*

12th November 2000 : How to spend winter with a heart ailment.

13th December 2000 : Winter Season — What to do? (Detailed discussion of effects of winter on the body and the precautions to be taken.)

14th January, 2001 : Sinusitis and Nasal Allergy. An informative lecture on this very common ailment.

11th February 2001 : Ayurvedic tips on heart ailments. A talk on all the ayurvedic drugs being used in heart disease.

14th March 2001 : Love and Intimacy — Know how to increase them? Dr. Chhajer discussed how to increase Love and Intimacy.

8th April 2001 : *Four Personality traits.* A detail discussion on set of characteristics which are natural to all individuals.

13th May 2001 : *What can we do in Summer?* ... asked one heart patient. Very useful tips for every one.

8th June 2001 : *Fear — the greatest enemy-I.* An informative lecture on how fear is introduced amongst the heart patients.

15th July 2001 : *Fear the greatest enemy-II.* Discussion on effects of fear and how to take care of it.

12th August 2001 : *How to analyse stress in daily life and take care.* Lecture included identification of stressors and their management.

9th September 2001 : *How to make up for daily walk, especially during the rainy season?* Detailed discussion on the various methods available which can replace conventional walking.

7th October 2001 : *How to make your spouse (married partner) happy?* Very useful tips for husbands and wives.

11th November 2001 : A delightful discussion was held on *How to enjoy Diwali with variety of sweets — Though you have a heart disease and Diabetes?* Demonstration was also given by our dietician on some types of sweets.

16th December 2001 : There was a talk by Dr. Chhajer on *how to build up new bridges and then how to maintain the old bridge.* Excellent response came from the participants.

13th January 2002 : Dr. Chhajer talked on a very interesting topic "Feng Shui" of present time.

10th February 2002 : Dr. Chhajer delivered a talk on Heart Attack and discussed the signs and symptoms of a heart attack? How to predict heart attack? And other things related to heart attack.

10th March 2002 : There was an extended discussion on details of oils, ghee etc. and *Which would be the best medium of cooking for the heart patients.*

7th April 2002 : There is so much stress, tension all around. In view of this, special lecture was given by Dr. Chhajer on *Meditation and Yoga for Heart.*

12th May 2002 : Exercise is very precious. Its effects on the heart and body were discussed by Dr. Chhajer.

9th June 2002 : Dr. Chhajer discussed on *Diabetic Self Care.* As majority of Heart Patients suffer from diabetes. A huge number of participants came and attended the lecture.

14th July 2002 : Heart Club Meeting was held on Bypass Surgery, Angioplasty and other so called invasive treatment of coronary Heart Disease.

11th August 2002 : One of the leading causes of heart disease and one of the major problems in this country was discussed. Dr. Chhajer delivered a lecture on causes and pattern of obesity in this country and its effective and practical management.

8th September 2002 : A very important discussion was made by Dr. Bimal Chhajer on "Heart". He discussed everything that one would like to know about this wonderful organ which keeps us alive.

Heart Talk magazine

This monthly journal, called *Heart Talk*, is a guide on life-style and update on non-invasive treatment. It is specially meant for heart patients or those who want to prevent heart disease. It has the latest knowledge on heart disease and its treatment.

Heart Talk was launched in October, 1998 and till now (Nov. 1999) about 42 issues have come out. *Heart Talk* is a twelve-page user friendly magazine. The magazine was released by Shri. Lal Krishan Advani, the then home minister of India.

The regular columns are Editorial, Patients' comments, the

Diet column, Latest research findings, New reviews, SAAOL's next camp dates, details of the heart club meetings in Delhi and so on.

I would recommend every heart patient and heart care enthusiast to subscribe to the *Heart Talk*.

Life membership for heart Talk Rs. 5000/-, for 5 years i.e. 60 issues Rs 1200/-, for 3 years i.e. 36 issues Rs. 800/- and 1 year (12 issues) is Rs 300/-)

SAAOL tea

Dr. Dean Ornish recommends no stimulants like coffee or tea for heart patients. Stimulants like caffeine, nicotine and other alkaloids are known to increase blood pressure, are not good for heart disease and are often addictive in nature.

I have seen many people addicted to tea and coffee. Because of the addiction, I could not convince them to stop these stimulant drinks. Many wanted just a hot drink.

On the advice of many known ayurveda and herb experts I gradually started recommending a herbal drink to heart patients which contains many heart friendly herbs and natural foods. The bark of the Arjun tree is one of the major components of this herbal drink. The taste improves by adding tulsi and some more herbs.

We ultimately named this drink the SAAOL tea or heart tea. In the last three years most of our patients reported additional benefits after consuming this tea. This tea is available at all our outlets.

"Understanding Heart Disease"

This book gives you detailed information about heart disease in simple language. More than 150 pages of this book are packed with information about heart disease, Dr. Dean Ornish, SAAOL etc. This is the best book for a patient for knowing and understanding his disease. This book is also available in Hindi.

"Food for Reversing Heart Disease"

This book is the outcome of four years of SAAOL's experiments with cooking. Whenever we cooked new food items in the series of hotels and resorts throughout India without oil we started putting all the recipes on paper. Our dieticians, gifted chefs in the hotels, our patients's family members all contributed recipes for this cookbook.

This book of about 500 pages has the theory of diet selection for heart patients and 200 hundred tasty recipes for cooking without a drop of oil. The book, an asset for heart patients, has recipes in both Hindi and English.

Food makes an important component of the SAAOL Heart Program and zero oil (visible oil) food is a certainly going to help in the reversal of heart disease. I would recommend this cooking method.

New Courses

1. SAAOL life-style courses for other lifestyle diseases:

A. High blood pressure

B. Diabetes

C. Obesity or overweight

D. Bronchial asthma

These courses have already started in 2003.

SAAOL Heart Program CD

In the era of computers and information technology we must use all the tools available to spread awareness on heart care.

SAAOL has developed a CD on its program. It demonstrates yoga, cooking techniques and three dimensional views of the heart's functioning.

Please keep in touch with us through our website and e-mail for the CD.

Best of luck

Remember : everything has a cause and effect relationship. If you work thoroughly and accurately there is every possibility that you will get the desired results. Of course there may be a factor called luck — but to my mind that is 5-10% contribution. I wish you that luck from my side. Just follow up and behave as if you are living a normal life — with health awareness.

You will definitely be successful.

Form for keeping in touch

SAAOL comes out with regular write ups and new information on heart care. Whenever new programs or books are launched you can be informed by post or e-mail.

Please fill up the following form and mail it to SAAOL at "SAAOL Heart Centre, 14/84 Vikram Vihar, Lajpat Nagar - IV, New Delhi - 110024".

Name ....

Age/Sex ....

Temporary Postal Address ....

....

Permanent Postal Address ....

....

Telephone: (R) : .... (O): ....

Fax: .... E-mail : ....

Profession: ....

....

Disease/Diagnosis, if any ....

....

Date: ....

Signature: ....

SAAOL Addresses

HEAD OFFICE : DELHI
14/84, Vikram Vihar,
Lajpat Nagar - IV, New Delhi — 110024.
Tel : 26235168, 26283098, 26211908
Fax : 26212016
E-mail : info@saaol.com
Website : www.saaol.com

BANGALORE OFFICE
25, S.P. Road, Off. 4th Temple Street
Malleswaram, Bangalore — 560003
Tel: 3462869

KOLKATA OFFICE
210/A, Rash Behari Avenue
Gariahat Crossing, Kolkata — 700029
Tel: 4641140 Fax: 4644449

CHENNAI OFFICE
566, Anna Salai
C/o Jeans Park India Pvt. Ltd.
Chennai — 600018
Tel: 4336435, 4337236

HYDERABAD OFFICE
4-i-7/A1/7/A King Kothi Road
Ramkote, Hyderabad — 500201
Tel: 4752232, 3224084

MUMBAI OFFICE
B - 301, Gold Mist
Thakur Complex, Kandivali (E)
Mumbai — 400101

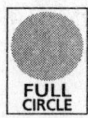

FULL CIRCLE

FULL CIRCLE publishes books on inspirational subjects, religion, philosophy, and natural health. The objective is to help make an attitudinal shift towards a more peaceful, loving, non-combative, non-threatening, compassionate and healing world.

FULL CIRCLE continues its commitment towards creating a peaceful and harmonious world and towards rekindling the joyous, divine nature of the human spirit.

Our fine books are available at all leading bookstores across the country.

FULL CIRCLE PUBLISHING

Registered Office
J-40, Jorbagh Lane, New Delhi 110003
Tel: 24620063, 24642762, 24642795 • Fax: 24645795
E-mail: fullcircle@vsnl.com / gbp@del2.vsnl.net.in

Bookstore
5B, Khan Market, New Delhi 110003
Tel: 24655641, 24655642

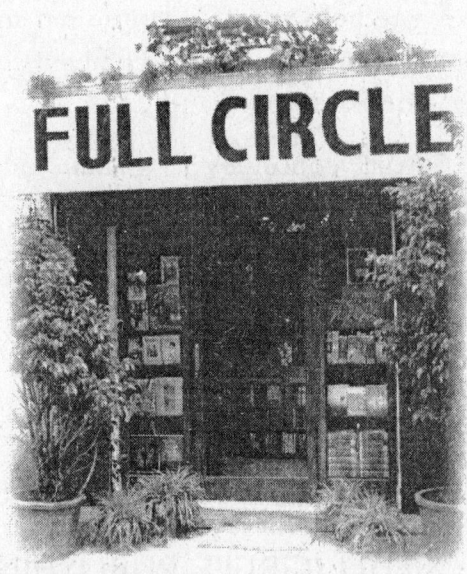
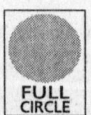

Join the

WORLD
WISDOM BOOK CLUB

Get the best of world literature in the
comfort of your home at fabulous
discounts!

Benefits of the Book Club

Wherever in the world you are, you can receive the best of
books at your doorstep.

- Receive FABULOUS DISCOUNTS by mail or at the
  FULL CIRCLE Bookstore in Delhi.

- Receive Exclusive Invitations to attend events being
  organized by **FULL CIRCLE**.

- Receive a FREE copy of the club newsletter — The World
  Wisdom Review — every month.

- Get UP TO 25% OFF.

Join Now!
It's simple. Just fill in the coupon overleaf and mail it to us at
the address below:

FULL CIRCLE
J-40, Jorbagh Lane, New Delhi 110003
Tel: 24620063, 24642762, 24642795 • Fax: 24645795

Yes, I would like to be a member of the
World Wisdom Book Club

Name ☐ Mr ☐ Mrs ☐ Ms _____

_____

Mailing Address _____

_____

_____

_____

City _____Pin_____

Phone _____ Fax _____

E-mail _____

Profession _____ D.O.B. _____

Areas of Interest _____

_____

Mail this form to:
The World Wisdom Book Club
J-40, Jorbagh Lane, New Delhi 110003
Tel: 24620063, 24642762, 24642795 • Fax: 24645795

REVERSAL OF HEART DISEASE